ENT Surgery and Disorders

06/06/2019

ENT Surgery and Disorders

with notes on nursing care and clinical management

A. J. INNES M B, B S, F R C S
Consultant Ear, Nose and Throat Surgeon,
United Norwich Hospitals

and

N. GATES SRN, DipN(London)
formerly Nursing Officer,
the Royal National Throat, Nose
and Ear Hospital, London

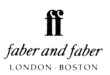

faber and faber
LONDON · BOSTON

First published in 1985
by Faber and Faber Limited
3 Queen Square, London WC1N 3AU

Typeset and printed in Great Britain by
Butler & Tanner Ltd, Frome and London
All rights reserved

British Library Cataloguing in Publication Data

Innes, A. J.

ENT surgery and disorders: with notes on
nursing care and clinical management.
1. Otolaryngology   2. Otolaryngological nursing
I. Title   II. Gates, N.
617'.51'0024613   RF45

ISBN 0-571-13653-2

Library of Congress Cataloging in Publication Data

Innes, A. J.

ENT surgery and disorders.
1. Otolaryngology, Operative.   2. Otolaryngological
nursing.   I. Gates, N.   II. Title.   [DNLM:
1. Otorhinolaryngologic Diseases—nursing.
2. Otorhinolaryngologic Diseases—surgery.   WV 168 158e]
RF51.156   1985   617'.51   85-1614

ISBN 0-571-13653-2 (pbk.)

Contents

Section Three – The Mouth and Throat

Acknowledgements

The authors extend their thanks to many colleagues who have helped in the preparation of this book. In particular Miss Gates is grateful to her former nursing colleagues at the Royal National Throat, Nose and Ear Hospital, London, while Mr Innes acknowledges his nursing and medical colleagues at the Norfolk and Norwich Hospital.

Mrs Merrilyn Crosskill SRN, a ward sister at the Norfolk and Norwich Hospital, has offered considerable advice and expertise for the nursing sections and both authors are extremely grateful to her.

Chapter 23 is included to remind nurses and doctors of the important part that the speech therapist, hearing therapist and social worker can play in the overall management and rehabilitation of patients with an ENT disorder. To Hilary Bumstead, Janet Lawrence and Betty Wise who contributed the respective sections, the authors' thanks are extended.

The text of the book has been greatly enhanced by line drawings and photographs. Mrs Audrey Besterman is warmly thanked for the superb drawings and for her patience in the preparing of them. To the Department of Medical Illustration, the Norfolk and Norwich Hospital and the Department of Clinical Photography, the Institute of Laryngology and Otology, London, who have helped with the photographs, thanks are also extended.

Figures 15/2a and 15/2b are included by permission of Richard Sellick FRCS, and Figure 15/3 is included by permission of Professor J.R. Moore, to both sources the authors and publishers extend their thanks.

Many people, both professional and lay, have helped with the 'putting together' of this book. In particular, Mr Innes acknowledges the painstaking typing and retyping of the manuscript by his wife. Both authors are indebted to Patricia Downie FCSP, Medical and Nursing Editor, Faber and Faber, for her constant support and encouragement throughout the preparation of this book.

Glossary

anosmia Loss of sense of smell

audiogram A test, using an audiometer, to measure hearing ability

audiometer A machine used to measure hearing ability

auriscope An instrument used to examine the ear, usually battery operated – a type of torch

bolus A lump of food chewed and ready to be swallowed

caloric test A method of testing the function of the vestibular system by irrigating the ear canal with warm and cold water respectively and then measuring the nystagmus produced

cholesteatoma A collection of squamous epithelium (skin) inside the middle ear cavity

CT scan A specialised type of radiographic examination to show structures in the body

decibel (dB) A unit of intensity of sound. A decibel is approximately the smallest possible change in sound intensity that can be detected by the human ear

diathermy A heating effect produced by passing a high frequency electric current through tissue(s). Used therapeutically to control bleeding (coagulation) or to divide tissue (cutting diathermy)

dysphagia Difficulty in swallowing

electrocochleography A type of hearing test. By using a very fine needle electrode placed through the ear drum tiny electrical impulses from the cochlea and auditory nerve can be recorded and measured. May be performed under a general anaesthesia. Particularly useful in children who are too young or incapable of co-operating with ordinary hearing tests

endolymph Fluid contained within the membranous labyrinth of the inner ear

endoscope An instrument used to carry out an endoscopy. It usually takes the form of a rigid metal tube with a source of bright light inside the tube but more recently endoscopes are becoming flexible (fibre-optic)

endoscopy The procedure whereby the interior of the hollow structures in the body is examined. The precise organ to be examined is usually indicated, e.g. laryngoscopy and oesophagoscopy are examinations of the larynx and oesophagus respectively

epistaxis A nose bleed

Eustachian tube (auditory tube) Connects nasopharynx and middle ear cavity. The tube opens by the muscular action associated with yawning or swallowing, and allows air to pass from the nasopharynx into the middle ear. It therefore keeps the middle ear at atmospheric pressure

epithelium Surface layer of tissue which covers the body or lines the hollow structures within the body

grommet (ventilation tube) A tiny tube which is usually made of a type of plastic, and which is inserted into the ear drum to equalise the pressure between the atmosphere and the middle ear

haematoma A collection of blood in the body tissues and outside the blood vessels. Usually occurs as a result of injury

hertz (Hz) A measurement of frequency of sound wave vibration (1 Hz = 1 cycle/second)

homograft A piece of tissue removed from a donor, often a cadaver, and transplanted into a recipient patient

iontophoresis A technique of anaesthetising the tympanic membrane

labyrinthitis Inflammation of the inner ear. If the vestibular apparatus only is involved the patient will be giddy, but if the cochlear is involved as well, deafness will result

ligate To tie. A term used in surgery, e.g. to tie a blood vessel to stop bleeding

meninges The three covering layers of the brain (dura, arachnoid, and pia). The dura is the thickest and toughest and lies against the bones of the skull cavity

metastasise Spread of malignant tumour from its primary site to a distant site by natural pathways, e.g. by lymphatics or the bloodstream

myringoplasty An operation to repair a perforation of the ear drum

myringotomy An incision in the ear drum through which fluid may be aspirated from the middle ear or a grommet inserted

nystagmus Movement of the eyes in a rhythmical manner – usually from side to side but may be up and down or rotatory

obturator A mechanical appliance for closing or occupying a hole or space, e.g. a type of dental plate to close the defect following the removal of part of the palate in a *maxillectomy*

otitis Inflammation of the ear. It may affect the outer ear (otitis externa) or middle ear (otitis media)

otosclerosis A condition which causes deafness. The stapes becomes fixed by the growth of new abnormal bone, and deafness results. It usually occurs in young adults, and may be familial

perilymph Inner ear fluid in which the membranous labyrinth is suspended within the bony labyrinth

phonation The production of purposive sound using the larynx

polyp A swelling with a stalk arising from mucous membrane or the body surface

presbycusis The deafness of ageing

prosthesis An artificial appliance to replace a part which has been lost or removed surgically

quinsy A peritonsillar abscess

raphe A fibrous line along which two muscles join

referred pain Pain which originates in a particular organ or structure which is felt in an area of skin supplied by the same nerve as the organ, e.g. pain which arises in the tonsil may be felt in the ear

speculum An instrument used in the inspection of a normally closed tube or passage. Specula vary in type according to their intended use. Many are tubular while others consist of two blades which are gently opened once the instrument has been inserted to allow inspection

sphincter A circle of muscle around an opening

stapedectomy An operation for the relief of otosclerosis. All or part of the stapes bone is removed and replaced by a piston, usually made of stainless steel or Teflon

tracheostomy An artificial opening made into the trachea through the neck

tracheotomy A surgical operation to make an opening from the exterior to the interior of the trachea

trismus Inability to open the mouth

Introduction

The letters ENT stand for ear, nose and throat. This book is concerned with some of the disorders of the ear, nose and throat and the authors hope it will provide an interesting general insight into the subject. Although the book is intended primarily for nurses, it will be of interest to other professionals whose work brings them into contact with patients suffering from ENT conditions.

No attempt has been made to give an *in-depth account* of nursing procedures, but nursing notes indicate the care and management which all nurses can use as the basis for nursing ENT patients. They should be supplemented with practical experience gained under supervision on an ENT unit. The book concentrates on ENT as it is encountered on general wards and in general hospitals. Specialised units dealing with the less common conditions are the exception and the special skills required on these units are beyond the scope of this book.

Unlike many other hospital departments the work of the ENT department is not divided into medical (with a physician) and surgical (with a surgeon). Instead the consultant who looks after patients suffering from ear, nose and throat conditions is usually called an ENT surgeon although he will look after both the medical and surgical aspects of ENT diseases. He does not do this work alone. As well as his medical colleagues in other specialties such as paediatrics, pathology, radiology and radiotherapy and oncology, he collaborates with nursing, physiotherapy, speech therapy, hearing therapy and social work colleagues. In addition, surgical operations may be carried out in combination with general, plastic, maxillofacial, and neuro- surgeons. The dental surgeon will be involved with some aspects of surgery of the maxilla, and similarly the thoracic surgeon may be involved with surgery to the oesophagus and trachea.

The reader will soon appreciate that ENT is not an isolated subject, and that the work of the ENT department can involve most departments in the hospital.

CHAPTER ONE

The ENT Outpatient Clinic

Patients with disease affecting the ears, nose or throat are frequently alarmed and confused by their symptoms. The family doctor may have prescribed treatment which has been only partly successful and consequently the patient has been referred for assessment by an ENT surgeon.

The patient should be brought into the consulting room by a nurse and should be greeted in a friendly, relaxed manner. Most young children will be shy and rather apprehensive so are best greeted with a smile and then ignored for a short while. If the child sees that the doctor is friendly towards his parents he will soon come to realise that he has nothing to fear and will probably co-operate in the examination.

After reading the letter of referral, the consultant will ask the patient for his own account of his symptoms. Additional information may then be obtained by asking relevant questions. Some patients will be precise in their account of symptoms while others will be less clear and will ramble on if given the chance. This only wastes time and they should kindly but firmly be reminded of the information being sought.

Details of past history, family history, current treatment and any allergies are recorded in the notes.

PHYSICAL EXAMINATION

Instruments used for examining the ear, nose and throat are, for the most part, quite different from the instruments used in other departments, and are designed specifically for the purpose (Fig. 1/1).

To examine most parts, bright light is essential. This is provided by an electric 'bull's-eye' lamp and is reflected towards the patient by means of a circular head mirror worn by the surgeon (Fig. 1/2).

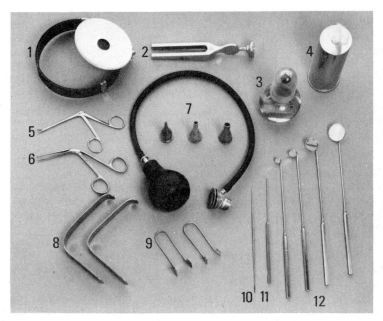

Fig. 1/1 Ear, nose and throat instruments. 1. Head mirror; 2. Tuning fork; 3. Spirit lamp; 4. Cotton-wool dispenser. 5. Cawthorne's aural forceps; 6. Tilley's dressing forceps; 7. Modified Siegle's otoscope with specula; 8. Lack's tongue depressors; 9. Thudicum's nasal specula; 10. Jobson-Horne wool carrier; 11. Wax hook; 12. Post-nasal and laryngeal mirrors

The delicate linings of the nose and throat and the skin of the ear canals are all sensitive, so must be handled very gently to avoid causing the patient any pain. When examining the nose it is often helpful to spray the nose with a mixture of local anaesthetic and adrenaline. This shrinks the lining of the nose and allows easier inspection of the nasal cavities.

The lower parts of the pharynx and the back of the nose are inaccessible to direct vision and are examined with the aid of a small mirror on a long handle (Fig. 1/2). To prevent the mirror from misting over, it should be warmed in the flame of a spirit lamp or in warm water. Before placing it in the patient's mouth the mirror must

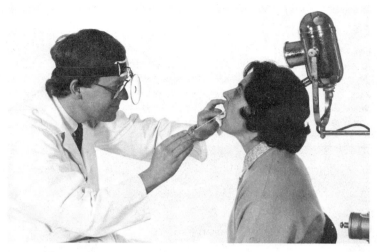

Fig. 1/2 Light from the 'bull's eye' lamp reflected from the circular head mirror worn by the surgeon

be tested on the back of the examiner's hand to see that it is not too warm.

Indirect laryngoscopy

This is a technique for examining the larynx. The patient sits upright in the chair, opens his mouth widely and protrudes his tongue as far as it will go. He is then instructed to breathe deeply and regularly through the open mouth. A piece of dry gauze is then wrapped around the tongue which is gently grasped by the surgeon: in this way the tongue can be coaxed out a little farther. The warmed mirror is then gently placed against the soft palate and the image of the larynx can be seen in the mirror.

Some patients will not tolerate mirror examination and will gag excessively. The throat may be sprayed with a small quantity of local anaesthetic such as 4% lignocaine or 5% cocaine. Spraying the throat will diminish or abolish the protective laryngeal reflexes, and patients should be warned not to eat or drink for three hours to avoid choking on food or aspirating fluid into the lungs. At all times the nurse should be on hand to reassure the patient and to steady the head if necessary. She should be ready to remove dirty instruments as necessary.

Ear examination

At times it may be necessary to examine the ears carefully and, at the same time, to remove any discharge which has accumulated. If it is convenient to use the operating microscope, the ear may be cleaned by suction (Fig. 1/3). Using specially designed instruments, fine manipulations may be performed.

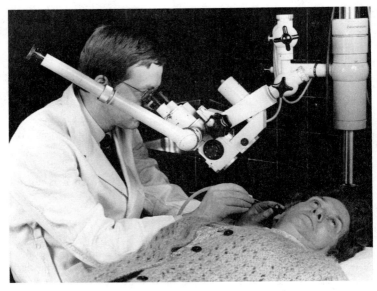

Fig. 1/3 Using the operating microscope to examine the ear

If the patient complains of deafness the hearing should be tested and tuning fork tests performed (see p. 37). The patient may be sent for an audiogram. If radiographic examination is required the necessary request form should give any relevant information.

Once the results of investigations are known the patient is seen again and the surgeon will discuss the diagnosis and any required treatment. Some minor procedures such as sinus washout, nasal polypectomy (sometimes), caloric testing, or more specialised hearing tests, may be carried out in the outpatient department, and these will be arranged for another visit. More major procedures will require admission.

It is well worth spending time explaining to the patient the nature of his or her symptoms in simple everyday language. This will avoid confusion and may save the patient unnecessary visits to his family doctor or to the clinic in the future.

Outpatient work is interesting and rewarding. As it is the first contact that most patients will have with the ENT department it is especially important that the patient is given the impression that it is well organised, kind and understanding. In all this the nurse has an important role.

CHAPTER TWO

The ENT Ward:
Applying the Nursing Process

The majority of patients who are admitted for ENT surgery are basically fit and mobile and will have an operation which will require them to remain in bed for only a short while afterwards. Such a patient's stay in hospital may be no more than two to three days.

For those patients undergoing major head and neck cancer surgery, more than one operation may be required and there may be a long period in hospital. The nursing skills required to cope with these two groups of patients are obviously very different.

The elderly and infirm comprise a third group of patients seen on ENT wards with significant medical problems for whom a sudden incident such as a severe nose bleed brings about their hospital admission. Many of these elderly patients may also be hard of hearing and the staff on the ENT ward must be particularly adept at dealing with the problems experienced by deaf patients, including the day to day care of hearing aids.

Although in an average busy ENT ward the majority of patients will be short stay they still require special skills to look after them and to ensure their safety while recovering from their operations. Even the so-called 'simple' operations, such as tonsillectomy, require the utmost vigilance in the postoperative recovery phase so that any complications, such as bleeding, may be spotted immediately and prompt action taken. Bleeding from the nose or throat or obstruction of the airway by blood or secretions in an unconscious patient are life-threatening situations. There is no excuse for complacency on the ENT ward.

THE NURSING PROCESS AND ITS APPLICATION TO ENT NURSING

Nurses must never lose sight of the fact that patients who come into hospital for surgery, investigation or treatment of a medical condition are people. They are not merely names, numbers or faceless beings.

Patients may be exposed to a considerable number of perhaps unpleasant or even undignified procedures and not surprisingly become very frightened. The method of planning nursing for patients called the 'Nursing Process' goes a long way towards treating patients as individuals and dispelling their fears.

The philosophy of the nursing process may be summarised thus:

1. Each patient is an individual needing individual care.
2. The patient and those closest to him should be involved in, and should have the chance to discuss, the care.
3. All levels of nursing staff should get together to assess the patient's needs and to plan the patient's nursing care.

In order to achieve this four stages of nursing care should be considered:

Assessment
Planning
Implementation
Evaluation

In ENT nursing many patients have very short stays in hospital for the more minor operations and the care plan involved is minimal, but for more extensive surgery the care needed is more complex and is planned for each individual.

First impressions are vitally important so when a patient is admitted to the ward, be it routine or an emergency, the nurse receiving the patient acts as an ambassador for the ward. The nurse should be seen to be welcoming, friendly and caring about the patient as an individual. If the patient is mobile he should be shown around the ward and introduced to fellow patients in the same room.

Assessment

Assessment commences from the moment the patient enters the ward. It will include individual nurse observations, as well as information from the patient together with anything relevant from his relatives and friends. Other members of the care team, e.g. the physiotherapist, dietitian, speech therapist, should be encouraged to add their observations where relevant.

This information is required:

(a) To establish what is normal for the individual patient.
(b) To identify specific problems and needs.
(c) To give the opportunity for the patient to ask questions.

(d) To provide a full history for all nursing staff to see.

Included in this assessment or nursing history will be questions relating to activities such as eating, sleeping, breathing habits, etc., as well as to the specific problems that has caused the patient to be admitted to hospital.

Planning

Planning the relevant care will be based on the information gathered. It will include goals to be achieved, and these should be from both the medical and nursing point of view so that all members of staff work in the same direction. Some goals may not always be totally achievable. Priorities should be decided and immediate needs dealt with promptly. Defining nursing problems and committing them to paper require skill and practice. *Good* planning almost always requires a multidisciplinary approach with all or some of the following being involved: physiotherapist, speech therapist, dietitian, hospital chaplain, radiographer, and community nursing services.

Implementation

In implementing the planned care, the nurses on duty will be allocated a group of patients; it is more satisfying to both patients and nurses if continuity can be achieved and the same nurses given the patients from whom they took the nursing history.

Obviously on a ward such as ENT, this is not always possible because of the large number of admissions and discharges each day. Whenever possible, senior nurses should work with junior nurses.

Before going to their patients the nurses should update the care plans, being aware of any changes in care or scheduled investigations or surgery. Where a change-over in the nursing shifts occurs, time should be made for open discussion so that any problems can be sorted out and *everyone* from the most junior upward has a chance to put forward their suggestions or point of view.

Evaluation

Evaluation is a continued form of assessment. It measures the effectiveness of implementation of the care plan and indicates to the nurse whether the individual patient is satisfied with the nursing care given and, hopefully, sees improvement.

Each stage of the nursing process is dependent upon the other, and at any stage re-assessment may have to be made and the evaluation on whether, by observation, the patient is better or worse.

At the centre of all this is an individual who wishes to keep his identity, to inter-relate with the nursing staff, who wish to help him cope with whatever has befallen him in an expert way that cannot be faulted, and who has a right to be involved in his care.

ADMITTING THE PATIENT

The patient's details should be carefully checked and recorded. This is part of the assessment phase of the nursing process although in some instances this will already have been done by the ward receptionist. Such details include:

Name
Address
Date of Birth
Religion
Name, address and telephone number of next of kin
Occupation

The patient's name, date of birth, hospital registration number and consultant's name are written on a wrist-band which is then securely fastened to the patient's wrist.

Details of current medication should be recorded and any drugs which the patient has brought in to hospital are collected for the doctor to see. Known allergies to drugs, to adhesive plaster or to any preparations which might be applied to the skin, such as iodine, must be noted in the records.

The nurse should weigh the patient and make sure that the weight is recorded in a prominent place on his treatment chart. The patient's weight is a vital piece of information because the dosage of many drugs, especially anaesthetic drugs, is critical and depends solely on the patient's weight.

The patient's blood pressure should be taken and recorded, and a specimen of urine tested for protein, sugar and blood, using the ward urine-testing sticks.

Explanation

Patients and, where appropriate, their relatives, should be told when the operation is due to be done, and given a time when it would be convenient to telephone after the operation. Where possible the patient should be given an idea of how long he will be in hospital after the operation.

Although the doctor will explain the details of the operation to the patient, the patient may well ask members of the nursing staff for such details; it is wiser to refer such questions either to the doctor or to a senior nurse on the ward. If the patient is given conflicting pieces of information by doctors and nurses on the same ward, he will quickly lose confidence. Obviously the ideal is for the nurse to be present when the doctor is explaining the operation to the patient, in that way she can reinforce the information given. This is an area which should be included in the nursing care plan.

If investigations, such as radiographic examinations, blood tests, or hearing tests, are required, they should be undertaken as soon as possible.

Anaesthesia

If the patient has been admitted for surgery he will be visited by the anaesthetist who will write-up the premedication.

The patient should have nothing to eat or drink for four to six hours before the planned time of operation. He should be told not to eat or drink and a notice saying 'Nil by mouth' should be attached to his bed or to the door of his room or both. It is highly dangerous to give an anaesthetic to a patient with a full stomach because he may vomit and inhale the vomit.

Planning the ward

On those days when there is an operating list, provision must be made for the fact that patients will require very close postoperative supervision (unless there is a recovery ward). Nurses will need to be available and the patient should be placed in such a position in the ward where he can be carefully observed.

The management of patients who have an ENT operation will depend to some extent on the specific operation performed. Such details will be found in the relevant chapters which follow.

PREPARING THE PATIENT FOR THEATRE

Whether the patient has been admitted for routine surgery or for emergency operation it is vital that the patient is received on to the ward by a friendly, efficient, and reassuring team of nurses and doctors. He must be absolutely confident that he is being looked after by people who know what they are doing.

As the time of operation approaches the nurse must be seen to take charge and, without losing any of her charm and friendliness, must put into action a series of events that ensures that the patient is safely delivered to the theatre for the correct operation.

1. The nurse must make sure the patient has had a bath and has been to the toilet. Patients who are due to have major surgery should have had a post-aural shave if requested and the hair washed. The patient wears only an operating gown but, depending on local policy, children may wear pyjamas.

2. The premedication drug should be checked carefully with a trained member of staff. Both nurses should then go to the patient and before giving the premedication the following points should be checked. (This is often conveniently accomplished using a check list which is then signed by the nurse and attached to the patient's notes.)

Check list

(a) Patient's nameband. The nurse should ask the patient his full name and check that it corresponds to the name on the wrist band, the patient's notes and the operating list.

(b) The consent form should have been signed and the patient should be aware of what operation he is going to have.

(c) The results of any blood tests asked for by the doctor must be available. If the results are abnormal, the doctor should be informed.

(d) If radiographs have been taken they must be available to be taken to the theatre.

(e) Does the next of kin know of the operation?

(f) All make-up, including nail varnish on fingers and toes, must be removed. This is to enable early cyanosis (blue colouration of the blood due to lack of oxygen) to be detected by looking at the colour of the nail bed.

(g) Any prostheses, for example an artificial limb, hair piece, or breast prosthesis (if a patient has had a mastectomy), should be removed.

(h) All jewellery should be removed and placed in safe keeping, with a receipt being given to the patient. If a ring cannot be removed it should be covered by adhesive tape.

(i) Dentures should be removed and placed in the patient's bedside locker. If the patient has any teeth which are crowned or loose this fact should be recorded prominently on the front of his notes. The anaesthetist and the surgeon should have been told this pre-operatively, but this reminder will ensure that they take particular care to protect these teeth during intubation.

(j) If the patient is to be lifted from his bed on to either a trolley to take him to the operating theatre or directly on to the operation table, he should be lying on a canvas.

(k) If the patient's bed is to go to the theatre, clean bed linen is essential.

(l) Cot sides should be securely fitted to the bed. These will help to prevent a confused or restless patient falling out of bed and injuring himself.

(m) The patient should be asked when he last had anything to eat or drink. For routine surgery he should have had nothing orally for at least four hours.

(n) Give the premedication drug (previously checked) as prescribed.

(o) Make sure that the patient understands that from the giving of the premedication he must not get out of bed in case he falls, because of the reaction of the premedication. The patient should be given a bell or buzzer so that he may summon help if required.

ON REACHING THE OPERATING THEATRE

The reception procedure in the operating theatre depends on local circumstances. If there is a patient reception area and designated reception nurses, the ward nurse formally hands over to her colleagues in reception. The full check list as above must have been completed to the satisfaction of the theatre staff.

If there are any queries these must be fully sorted out by the ward nurse before she leaves the patient and returns to the ward.

In some hospitals the ward nurse will accompany the patient into the anaesthetic room. Although the patient may have had a sedative premedication he may still be anxious and will look to the nurse for reassurance. A little light conversation is usually all that is required – just enough to keep the patient relaxed and his mind occupied until the anaesthetist arrives.

The anaesthetist may ask the nurse to help, for example by taking the patient's arm out of the operating gown so that the blood pressure cuff can be put on. The nurse may be asked to gently squeeze the patient's arm in order to distend the veins. This makes it much easier to give the intravenous injection of the anaesthetic drugs. Once this has been done and the patient is asleep the nurse will be thanked and may return to the ward.

CHAPTER THREE

The ENT Operating Theatre

Having looked at the generalities of the outpatient examination and the ward, let us now move into the surgical environment.

In many respects ear, nose and throat surgery differs from some of the other branches of surgery. Many of the structures operated on are very small and the access to them may be restricted, for example, the structures of the middle ear are tiny and difficult to get at via the ear canal. Specially designed fine instruments have to be used (Fig. 3/1). In order to work safely and precisely the surgeon must be able to see exactly what he is doing, and so good *lighting* is

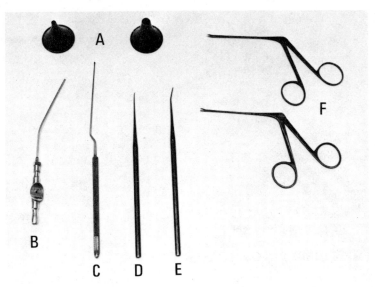

Fig. 3/1 Ear surgery instruments. A. Ear specula; B. Sucker; C. Myringotomy knife; D. Hughes' mobiliser; E. Rosen elevator; F. Middle ear forceps

vital. With the exception of operations done on the neck, for example laryngectomy, the illumination provided by the overhead operating light in the operating theatre is usually inadequate. The surgeon therefore wears a headlight (Fig. 3/2) which directs a narrow beam of bright light on to the operative field, such as the nose or mouth.

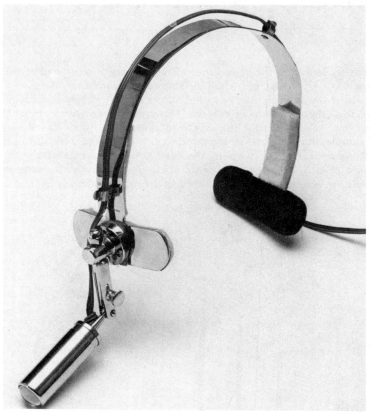

Fig. 3/2 Operating headlight

THE OPERATING MICROSCOPE

Many of the recent advances in middle ear surgery would not have been possible without the operating microscope. This provides a magnified, highly illuminated view of the structures to be operated on.

The microscope has two eyepieces so that the operator has binocular vision and sees things in three dimensions. There is also a teaching side-arm so that interested onlookers may see the operation being performed and surgeons in training may be shown how to perform the operation (Figs. 3/3 and 3/4).

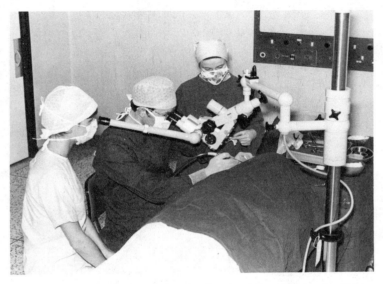

Fig. 3/3 The operating microscope showing the side-arm through which an onlooker may watch, and receive instruction

The operating microscope has other uses, namely for microsurgery of the larynx, for removal of the pituitary gland (hypophysectomy) and, by some surgeons, for certain nasal operations such as nasal polypectomy.

ANAESTHESIA

The majority of ear, nose and throat operations, are performed under general anaesthesia. Before a general anaesthetic is given it is common practice to give a premedication drug. Sedative drugs have the effect of reducing anxiety and pain if these are present and produce a degree of sedation which allows a smooth induction of the

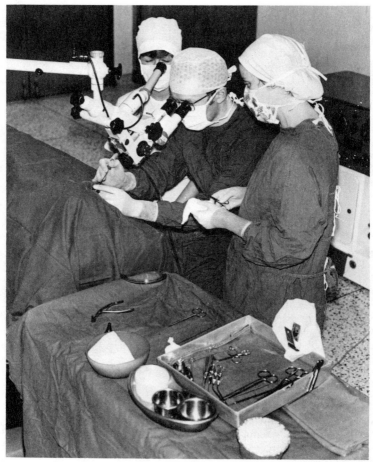

Fig. 3/4 The operating microscope and positioning of the instrument tray

anaesthetic. Drugs commonly used for this purpose are papaveretum (Omnopon) and pethidine.

It is also a great advantage, especially when an operation on the mouth or throat is planned, to reduce salivary secretion. Atropine or hyoscine are useful in this respect. Atropine and atropine-like drugs also have the advantage of eliminating the bradycardia (slowing of the heart) which results when the vagus nerve is stimulated. This is particularly important in some throat operations because there is a rich innervation by the vagus nerve around the larynx and pharynx.

The premedication drugs are usually given by injection but some anaesthetists prefer simply to give drugs such as diazepam or lorazepam to relieve anxiety, and these may be given orally. For children undergoing a routine operation such as tonsillectomy the sedative premedication drug may be omitted and the child given atropine in syrup form.

For most operations general anaesthesia begins with its induction using an injection of a short-acting barbiturate such as thiopentone and a short-acting muscle relaxant such as suxamethonium (Scoline). An endotracheal tube of appropriate size for the patient is passed via the mouth or nose into the larynx. The endotracheal tube is then connected to the anaesthetic machine and the patient kept anaesthetised by breathing a mixture of nitrous oxide, oxygen and a volatile agent such as halothane. By placing an endotracheal tube through the larynx, blood and other secretions are prevented from passing into the trachea and lungs.

In young children the region of the larynx directly below the vocal cords (the cricoid region) is the narrowest part of the upper airway and is circular. By selecting an endotracheal tube of the correct size, calculated from the child's age, a snug fit is ensured and aspiration of blood prevented. In adults, however, the narrowest part of the airway is at the level of the vocal cords; this is wedge-shaped rather than circular so the endotracheal tube is fitted with an inflatable cuff which goes beyond the cords and into the upper trachea. After the tube has been passed the cuff is inflated to produce an airtight seal.

For longer operations the patient may be given a paralysing drug such as curare, which leaves the respiratory muscles paralysed and the patient unable to breathe for himself. In such cases the endotracheal tube is connected to a mechanically operated ventilating machine which takes over the patient's respiration until the effects of the curare wear off, or the drug neostigmine is given to reverse its action at the end of the operation.

For short operations where there is to be no surgical intervention in the mouth, nose or throat and therefore no risk of bleeding and inhalation of blood, the endotracheal tube may be dispensed with and the anaesthetist will hold a mask over the patient's nose and mouth while he breathes a mixture of halothane, nitrous oxide and oxygen.

If the surgeon wishes to examine the larynx under a general anaesthetic and perhaps to take biopsies from a vocal cord tumour, he
may prefer to do this without an endotracheal tube in situ. In this
case, once the patient has been anaesthetised and the surgeon has
positioned the laryngoscope (see p. 151), the patient will be kept
anaesthetised by further intravenous injections of thiopentone and
Scoline while the respiration is maintained by a high pressure jet of
oxygen delivered through a fine bore needle attached to the laryngoscope.

Safe and successful anaesthesia depends on giving the correct
amount of the right drug. The correct dose is calculated from the
knowledge of the patient's weight and this is especially important
when anaesthetising children. This is the reason why the patient
should be accurately weighed before an operation and the *correct*
weight prominently recorded in his notes and on the anaesthetic
sheet.

Local anaesthesia
It is difficult even to see into a normal nose but if there is a lot of
bleeding it may become almost impossible to see what is happening.
Under such circumstances operating is difficult and even dangerous.
Applying vasoconstrictors, such as cocaine, to the nasal mucosa will
shrink the blood vessels. Not only is the amount of bleeding reduced
to a minimum but the actual thickness of the mucosa is reduced so
allowing a better view of the nose.

It is therefore highly desirable for most nasal operations to be
performed under general anaesthesia with some form of *local* anaesthetic to provide vasoconstriction. The local anaesthetic may be applied by the surgeon or the anaesthetist before the patient is taken
into the operating theatre in order to give the maximum time for the
vasoconstrictor to work. This may take the form of 25% cocaine
paste painted around the inside of the nose. Alternatively the cocaine
paste may be applied after the patient has been anaesthetised and
taken into theatre.

Some operations such as antral washout or removal of small
numbers of nasal polypi are frequently carried out using only local
anaesthesia. The mucous membrane of the nose and throat is per-
meable to solutions of local anaesthetic so the lining of the nose or
throat may be anaesthetised effectively by using either cotton wool
or ribbon gauze soaked in a local anaesthetic solution. The excess
solution is then wrung out and the damp wool or gauze applied to

the area to be anaesthetised and is left for at least 10 minutes. Alternatively, the solution may be simply sprayed into the nose or throat.

Anaesthetising the tympanic membrane is more difficult because the ear drum is covered by a layer of squamous epithelium which is relatively impermeable to a solution of local anaesthetic applied directly to it.

IONTOPHORESIS
A technique known as iontophoresis has been developed in which a solution of a local anaesthetic is placed in the ear canal and a small electric current passed through the solution. This has the effect of driving the local anaesthetic into the tympanic membrane and so anaesthetising the ear drum. Procedures such as myringotomies may then be performed in the outpatient clinic.

Hazards of local anaesthesia

The use of local anaesthetic agents such as cocaine is not without its dangers and great care must be taken. Before giving a patient cocaine, or indeed any drug, a thorough history of drug allergies should be taken. If the patient is allergic to cocaine even a small amount of the drug will give rise to an *anaphylactic reaction* and the patient may collapse with a weak thready pulse and a low or even unrecordable blood pressure. The skin will feel cold and clammy and the patient will be cyanosed. This is a medical emergency and help must be summoned immediately. Full resuscitation facilities must be available. The patient should be laid flat, given oxygen, and all tight clothing should be loosened. An intravenous infusion should be available.

Alternatively the patient may, inadvertently, be given too much cocaine, or he may have swallowed the cocaine solution into the stomach where it is absorbed into the bloodstream much more quickly. For this reason patients must be told *never* to swallow the cocaine solution but to spit out any solution into a bowl or paper tissues. For an adult, the maximum recommended dose of cocaine is 200mg (the amount contained in 2ml of a 10% solution). If more than this is given the patient may become restless and agitated and may have a convulsion.

Some patients however will have a vasovagal attack and will faint. Though the skin may be pale and clammy, the pulse is usually slow and strong. The patient should be laid flat and the legs should be elevated. The patient will usually quickly recover from a vasovagal attack but it is wise to abandon any thoughts of continuing the procedure under local anaesthesia.

ROLE OF THE NURSE IN THE OPERATING THEATRE

Having indicated that ear, nose and throat surgery differs from other branches of surgery, how does it differ for the nurse?

Many of the operations are performed by the surgeon through small dark holes and although the surgeon knows what he is doing, it is quite likely that nobody else will – because they cannot see the operative field. This includes the nurse. It is therefore of the utmost importance that the nurse who is scrubbed is thoroughly familiar with the operation being performed.

The nurse can anticipate the instruments, equipment or dressings that will be required. As the surgeon finishes using one instrument and puts it down, the new instrument should be available and placed into his hand *in the correct position* for immediate use. The last thing a surgeon wants is to have to keep looking away from the operative field to search for an instrument, or to be handed an instrument the wrong way up or pointing in the wrong direction, just as he has reached a vital or delicate stage in the proceedings. A rapport between surgeon and nurse will enable difficult procedures to be accomplished swiftly, easily and safely.

Many surgeons have likes and dislikes regarding instruments, sutures, dressings, etc. It is helpful for a nurse to keep some sort of card index on which these individual whims are recorded.

Patients are usually nursed in the semi-prone position, and if surgery has been performed in the mouth or throat and there is a risk of bleeding, e.g. tonsillectomy, the foot of the bed is elevated slightly. This ensures that if there is any bleeding the blood will flow out of the mouth and nose away from the larynx thus minimising the dangers of inhalation.

Following tracheostomy or laryngectomy, suction must be immediately available at all times so that blood and secretions may be gently but thoroughly removed from the mouth, pharynx, nose or trachea. In addition to suction tubing there should be a selection of flexible suction catheters as well as more rigid pharyngeal suckers.

Oxygen must always be instantly available together with a selection of face masks.

In patients who are recovering from anaesthesia and who are not yet fully conscious there is a tendency for the tongue to fall backward causing respiratory obstruction. To prevent this happening a rubber or plastic airway will have been placed in the mouth by the anaesthetist and the patient's chin may need to be held forward in order to maintain the airway.

The recovery room nurse

Once the operation has been completed there is much to do. The patient who is recovering from a general anaesthetic will not yet have regained his life-preserving laryngeal reflexes and will be at risk from airway obstruction and inhalation of blood or other secretions. The immediate care of the patient is assumed by the anaesthetist; once he is satisfied that the patient is sufficiently conscious to protect his own airway, the patient is then transferred to the recovery area to the care of trained nurses. At this point the anaesthetist or a member of the theatre staff explains to these nurses the nature of the operation performed and whether there are any drains or packs in situ.

It is the duty of the recovery nurse to:

1. Maintain the patient's airway. Respirations should be regular and this may be confirmed by observation of the chest movement. Listen carefully to the sound of the breathing, which should be regular. Secretions or blood in the airway sound 'rattly'. If there is any difficulty in keeping the airway open as shown by the patient's breathing becoming obstructed, by the development of stridor (see p. 136) or by development of cyanosis, expert help should be summoned immediately. In a well-equipped recovery area, by each patient's bed, there will be an emergency button to call help.
2. Perform regular checks and record pulse and blood pressure.
3. Watch carefully for any signs of bleeding such as fresh blood appearing at the nose or mouth or of excessive swallowing by the patient. The surgeon should be informed immediately.

In the recovery area there will be a fully equipped resuscitation trolley, and everyone who works in the recovery area must know where all the emergency equipment is kept and how the equipment works.

POSTOPERATIVE ANALGESIA

Many operations are associated with a greater or lesser degree of postoperative pain or discomfort. To minimise this the anaesthetist will usually prescribe some postoperative analgesia which usually takes the form of an opiate injection, e.g. papaveretum.

This analgesia is usually given just as the patient is waking up and, hopefully, before he becomes agitated. The dose is carefully checked by two nurses and given intramuscularly. Following the injection the patient settles into a contented sleep from which he may be easily roused. Patients should be allowed to recover from their operation in peace and quiet while being carefully and expertly observed. They should not be shaken or shouted at just to see if they are awake.

Before leaving the recovery area the patient should be seen by the anaesthetist. Provided the patient's condition is satisfactory he may then be taken back to the ward, by a nurse and a porter.

RETURNING TO THE WARD

The journey to the ward is potentially hazardous and there must be adequate facilities for resuscitating the patient if the need arises. The bed or trolley must be able to be easily tipped head down in case the patient vomits or if there is any sign of bleeding. Portable suction, usually in the form of a foot-operated pump, must accompany each patient, together with connecting tubing and a suitable pharyngeal sucker. There should also be an airway and a gag to open the mouth.

On arrival at the ward the patient is then transferred to the care of the nurse in charge, giving full details of the operation, whether there are any drains or packs and any instructions for their management. Details of postoperative analgesia and/or other drugs given and any intravenous infusion, should be clearly given. The patient's notes, including notes of the operation, should accompany the patient at all times. Once the ward nurse is satisfied with the patient's condition the recovery nurse will return.

The patient who has returned from the operating theatre should be placed in such a position in the ward that he can be observed at all times by members of the nursing staff. The type of postoperative care and management will depend not only on the type of operation performed but also on the wishes of the surgeon. Specific nursing care will be indicated in the relevant chapters throughout the book.

Section One – The Ear

CHAPTER FOUR

Anatomy and Physiology

The ear may be described in three parts (Fig. 4/1):
1. The outer ear
2. The middle ear
3. The inner ear

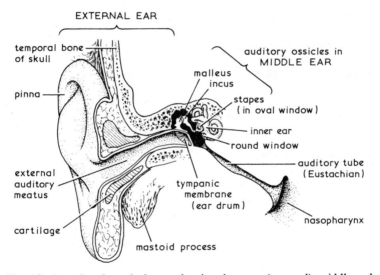

Fig. 4/1 A section through the ear showing the outer (external), middle and inner ear

OUTER OR EXTERNAL EAR

The outer ear protects the more delicate middle and inner ear structures. It consists of the *pinna* and the *external ear canal*.

The pinna is composed of flexible cartilage covered on both sides by thin skin. The shape and size of the pinna is variable. The external ear canal is a blind pit lined by skin at the bottom of which lies the *tympanic membrane*. The canal should be considered in two parts:

1. The *outer third* of the canal is supported by cartilage which is continuous with the cartilage of the pinna. It is lined by thick skin containing hair follicles and wax glands.
2. The *inner two-thirds* is supported by bone and the skin lining is very thin with no hair follicles or wax glands.

The ear canal is not a straight tube but is slightly bent. While this further minimises the risk of damage to the middle and inner ear by direct trauma it also means that when it becomes necessary to examine the tympanic membrane, the tube has to be straightened. This is done by gently pulling the pinna upward and backward.

Tympanic membrane (ear drum) (Fig. 4/2)

The tympanic membrane is neither flat, nor round and is not set at right angles to the ear canal.

The drum is shaped like a very shallow cone: the vertical height is slightly greater than the width, and the surface of the drum faces downward and forward.

Most of the tympanic membrane is three layers thick. The *outer layer* is squamous epithelium continuous with the skin of the ear canal. The *inner layer* is mucous membrane which lines the middle

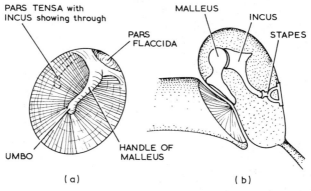

Fig. 4/2 The tympanic membrane (ear drum). (a) As seen using an auriscope; (b) In cross-section

ear cleft. The *middle layer* lying between the two is formed of fibrous tissue, the fibres of which are arranged radially, like the spokes of a wheel, radiating from the centre of the tympanic membrane, the *umbo*. This fibrous layer gives the tympanic membrane its support and this part of the ear drum is called the *pars tensa*. The handle of the *malleus* bone is actually embedded in the pars tensa. Around the rim of the tympanic membrane the fibrous layer is condensed to form a ring like the rim of a wheel. This is called the fibrous *annulus* and fits into a groove in the bone, the *bony annulus*.

The upper part of the tympanic membrane lacks the fibrous middle layer and so is less well supported than the pars tensa. This is the *pars flaccida*.

The outer skin layer of the tympanic membrane resembles skin elsewhere on the body inasmuch as the skin cells are constantly being shed and replaced by new cells. There is therefore a constant migration of skin cells from the region of the umbo towards the edge of the tympanic membrane and then along the ear canal where they mix with the wax and are shed to the outside.

The migration of skin cells is particularly important when *cholesteatoma* is considered later (see p. 56).

MIDDLE EAR (Fig. 4/3)

This is an air-containing cavity situated in the temporal bone. The actual middle ear cavity forms part of the middle ear cleft. This consists of the *Eustachian tube*, the *middle ear cavity* and the *mastoid air cell* system and is important when pathological conditions of the middle ear, such as acute otitis media, are discussed in subsequent chapters. (If you take a piece of plasticine about the size of a pea and squash it between thumb and forefinger, that will give you some idea of the size and shape of the middle ear cavity.)

The lateral wall of the middle ear is convex inward and is formed by the tympanic membrane. The gap between medial and lateral walls, which is only about 1mm in the region of the umbo, is bridged by three tiny bones (the *ossicles*) - known as the *malleus, incus* and *stapes*.

The handle of the malleus is embedded in the pars tensa of the tympanic membrane and can be easily seen when the ear is examined with an auriscope. The head of the malleus is situated at a higher level in the uppermost recess of the middle ear called the *attic*. In the attic the head of the malleus articulates with the body of the

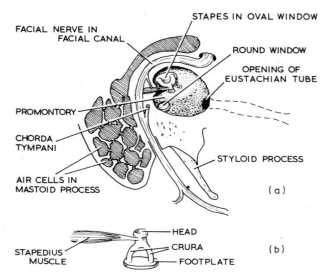

Fig. 4/3 The middle ear. (a) Showing the relationship of other structures; (b) Showing the stapes in detail

incus by means of a joint with a joint capsule. Another joint is located between the slender long process of the incus with the head of the smallest bone in the body, the stapes.

The stapes is shaped like a stirrup, and two slender limbs, the *crura*, connect the head with the footplate. The footplate is oval in shape and fits into an opening on the medial wall of the middle ear, the *oval window*.

Sound waves passing down the ear canal cause the tympanic membrane to vibrate. This vibration is then transmitted across the ossicular chain to the footplate of the stapes. Each time the footplate moves, the inner ear fluids are set into vibration and small electrical impulses are generated in the organ of hearing, the *cochlea*. These electrical impulses are then transmitted along the VIIIth (cochlear) cranial nerve to the brain where they are translated into meaningful sound.

Fluids are not compressible so there must be some mechanism to prevent the pressure from rising within the delicate inner ear. Each time the footplate of the stapes moves inward at the oval window, there is a corresponding outward movement of the inner ear membrane at the *round window*, and vice versa.

Two tiny muscles are attached to the ossicular chain to prevent them from moving unduly in response to loud noise and from damaging the inner ear. These are the *tensor tympani*, whose tendon is attached to the neck of the malleus and the *stapedius* which attaches to the neck of stapes.

The medial wall of the middle ear bulges in towards the middle ear cavity. This bulge is called the *promontory* and is caused by the underlying cochlea.

The *facial* (VIIth cranial) nerve supplies the muscles of facial expression and runs a tortuous course through the temporal bone. The facial nerve enters the apex of the temporal bone at the *internal auditory meatus* alongside the auditory nerve and the vestibular nerve. It then passes laterally until it reaches the middle ear cavity. Here it turns backward and runs along the medial wall of the middle ear across the top of the oval window. It then makes another turn around the oval window and passes directly downward in the bony partition between the middle ear and the mastoid. When it nears the bottom of the mastoid process it leaves the skull, turns forward and runs through the parotid gland to reach the muscles of the face.

The facial nerve is at risk of damage in any ear operation. After an ear operation *every* patient should be carefully looked at to check that the facial nerve is undamaged. If damage is suspected, the *surgeon who performed the operation should be notified* immediately.

Another nerve, the *chorda tympani* nerve, crosses the tympanic membrane like the chord of a circle, carrying taste fibres from the anterior two-thirds of the tongue. This nerve is often damaged during ear surgery and may give rise to temporary symptoms of disturbance of taste.

It is convenient to mention here the *Eustachian (auditory) tube* which passes upward from the nasopharynx to the middle ear. Its function is to allow air to enter the middle ear cavity and to equalise the pressures between the middle ear and the surrounding atmosphere. This is essential if the middle ear sound conducting mechanism is to function properly.

The tube is lined with mucous membrane and is usually closed. It is opened by the action of small muscles attached to the palate which come into action during swallowing or yawning.

In the infant and young child, the Eustachian tube is relatively shorter, wider, and more nearly horizontal than in the adult. These anatomical differences are partly responsible for the fact that children are more prone to attacks of ear infection than adults.

INNER EAR

The inner ear houses the organ of hearing, the *cochlea* and the organ of balance, the *vestibule*.

Cochlea (Fig. 4/4)

The cochlea is so called because it resembles a snail's shell. Its structure is complicated but can be made easier to understand if it is thought of as two and a half turns of a spiral stretched out to make one long tapering tube.

This tube is located in the densest part of the temporal bone, the petrous temporal bone. The tube is further subdivided into three compartments by two delicate membranes running lengthwise.

The upper compartment, the *scala vestibuli*, connects directly with the oval window containing the stapes footplate. The scala vestibuli contains clear, colourless fluid known as *perilymph* which resembles cerebrospinal fluid in its chemical composition. The lower compartment, known as the *scala tympani*, ends at the round window membrane and contains perilymph. These upper and lower compartments are in direct communication at the distal end of the cochlea.

The middle compartment, the *scala media*, contains fluid known as *endolymph* whose chemical composition is quite different from the perilymph.

Within the scala media lies the *organ of Corti*. This collection of specialised cells sits on the basilar membrane and runs the whole length of the cochlea. It is in the organ of Corti that the most important function of the cochlea is carried out. Sound waves which cross the middle ear as vibrations of the ossicular chain are converted into electrical impulses which may then travel along the auditory nerve to the brain.

As the stapes footplate moves, a pressure wave travels through the scala vestibuli and scala tympani, causing movements of the basilar membrane and of the hair cells situated in rows along its length. The hairs on each hair cell are embedded in the gelatinous *tectorial membrane*, and as the hair cells themselves move the tips of the hairs are kept stationary. This causes the hairs to bend and this bending

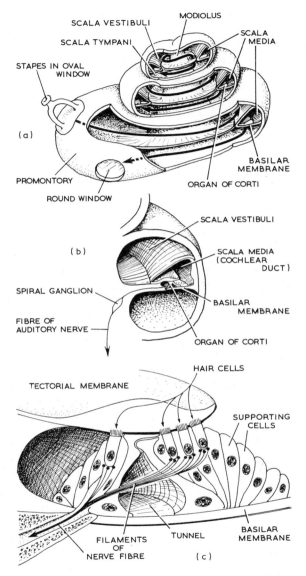

SCALA VESTIBULI

MODIOLUS

SCALA TYMPANI

SCALA MEDIA

STAPES IN OVAL WINDOW

(a)

BASILAR MEMBRANE

PROMONTORY

ORGAN OF CORTI

ROUND WINDOW

SCALA VESTIBULI

(b)

SCALA MEDIA (COCHLEAR DUCT)

SPIRAL GANGLION

BASILAR MEMBRANE

FIBRE OF AUDITORY NERVE

ORGAN OF CORTI

HAIR CELLS

TECTORIAL MEMBRANE

SUPPORTING CELLS

BASILAR MEMBRANE

FILAMENTS OF NERVE FIBRE

TUNNEL

(c)

Fig. 4/4 The cochlea. (a) Cut away to show fluid compartments; (b) Cross-section through a single turn; (c) The organ of Corti in detail

generates a tiny electrical impulse within the hair cells. The electrical impulses are gathered together in the nerve filaments and are then relayed along the auditory nerve.

For the sake of compactness, the tubular structure of the cochlea is wound two and a half times round a central pillar of bone, the *modiolus*. The first turn of the cochlea is wider than the other, and bulges into the medial wall of the middle ear where we see it as the promontory.

The vestibule

The maintenance of posture and balance is a complex matter in which certain parts of the brain, notably the cerebellum, continually process information coming from various sources. These sources include the eyes, the proprioceptors in skin, joints and muscles and the vestibular system. These systems work in harmony and normal balance may be seriously impaired by a defect in any one of these systems.

The vestibule consists of a series of interconnecting cavities and tunnels in the bone. This is collectively known as the bony labyrinth and contains the fluid perilymph. Suspended in the perilymph is a membranous bag which mimics the shape of the bony labyrinth but which contains the fluid endolymph and is known as the *membranous labyrinth*.

There are three parts to the vestibular labyrinth, namely the *semicircular canals*, the *saccule* and the *utricle* (Fig. 4/5). They have slightly different functions but may be considered together.

The sensory receptors in the labyrinth are responsible for converting physical factors, namely movements of the head, into nervous impulses which then travel in the vestibular nerve to the brain.

The sensory receptors consist of hair cells whose fine hairs are embedded in a membrane. As the head starts to move or turn, the inner fluids tend to try and remain in the same place as a result of their inertia. This then causes a distortion of the hair which results in the generation of nerve impulses. In the resting state there is a regular stream of impulses generated in the vestibule but as the vestibular hair cells are stimulated by movement the rate of impulses changes.

The important thing to realise is that in response to movements of the head, the information transmitted to the brain is equal and opposite from the two labyrinths. The impulses effectively cancel each other out.

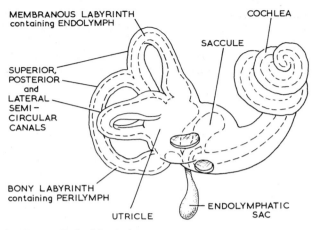

MEMBRANOUS LABYRINTH
containing ENDOLYMPH

COCHLEA

SACCULE

SUPERIOR,
POSTERIOR
and
LATERAL
SEMI -
CIRCULAR
CANALS

BONY LABYRINTH
containing PERILYMPH

UTRICLE

ENDOLYMPHATIC
SAC

Fig. 4/5 The vestibular labyrinth

One way to think of this is to imagine a man rowing a boat. As long as he pulls equally with both oars the boat will go in a straight line. As soon as the pull becomes unequal, either by pulling harder with one oar, or by stopping rowing with one oar, the boat will go round in circles. So it is in the ear. If as a result of disease or some abnormal physical stimulation the impulses from each side become unbalanced, the patient will experience a false sensation of movement. This is termed *vertigo* (see Chapter 9).

The three semicircular canals are placed at right angles to one another, each in a separate plane, and the ends of each canal open into the utricle. They are termed superior, posterior and lateral (Fig. 4/5). By this means turning movements of the head in any direction may be detected.

Each canal consists of a C-shaped tube with a swelling, the *ampulla*, at one end. The sensory receptor is located within the ampulla and is known as a *christa*. Each sensory receptor works on the hair-cell principle described earlier.

The membranous duct of the cochlea (scala media) and the saccule, the semicircular canals of the utricle, all contain endolymph. The saccule and the utricle are joined by the Y-shaped endolymphatic duct. The end of this duct is expanded to form the endolymphatic sac which lies between the two layers of the dura on the posterior surface of the petrous temporal bone.

Although this may seem complicated it *is* relevant. In the condition known as Ménière's disorder there is excessive production of endolymph. The unpleasant symptoms of this disorder may be alleviated by draining the excess fluid, and this may be achieved by locating the endolymphatic sac and opening it to allow the excess fluid to drain away (saccus decompression).

CHAPTER FIVE

Deafness: Hearing Aids:
Effects of Noise

While most of us take for granted the ability to hear well there are many people whose hearing is impaired, and this imposes on them a great social handicap.

Any factor which interferes with the transmission of sound from the outer ear, through the middle and inner ear and along the auditory pathway to the brain, will result in defective hearing or deafness (Fig. 5/1).

If there is interference with the conduction of sound along the ear canal, through the tympanic membrane and the chain of ossicles as far as the footplate of the stapes, the resultant deafness is known as *conductive deafness.*

If there is a defect within the sense organ of hearing (cochlea) or the nerve of hearing, the deafness is known as *sensori-neural* or *perceptive.*

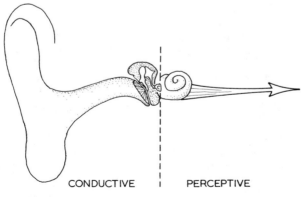

CONDUCTIVE   PERCEPTIVE

Fig. 5/1 Types of deafness

CLINICAL ASSESSMENT FOR DEAFNESS

Any patient who complains of impaired hearing should be questioned carefully and patiently regarding his hearing difficulties. He should be asked whether one or both ears are affected; did the deafness come on suddenly or develop slowly; has there been any pain in the ears or discharge; does he notice any abnormal noises in the ear – hissing, ringing, humming, etc. (i.e. tinnitus); and has there been any disturbance of balance? The patient's present and/or past occupation(s) should be recorded and he should be asked specifically if there has been any exposure to loud noise. Other things to be recorded include any family history of deafness, a drug history, whether there has been any previous ear surgery or any symptoms of nasal disease. The ears are then examined clinically.

Examination

The external ears are inspected first for any abnormality, e.g. congenital absence of the pinna, and the skin around the pinna examined for any scars associated with previous surgery. The ear canals are inspected to make sure that they are free from wax, debris or discharge, and then the tympanic membrane is examined. If the patient appears to have a middle ear effusion, particular attention is paid to the nose and nasopharynx since any disease process which interferes with the function of the Eustachian tube may give rise to secretory otitis media (see p. 51).

Hearing tests

The hearing may then be tested clinically. In order to avoid the patient's lip-reading, the tester should hide his mouth from the patient either by covering it with his hand or a piece of card, or alternatively he should stand behind the patient. It is better to test each ear separately, so it is necessary to keep the other ear occupied. This process is called 'masking', and is simply achieved by rubbing a flat piece of paper against the ear not being tested.

The examiner then speaks in a loud conversational voice, a quiet voice or a whisper, and records the distance at which the patient can correctly repeat what the examiner says. The results may then be simply recorded in the notes, e.g. (R) ear – whispered voice 3 feet; (L) ear – loud voice 2 feet, giving a valuable indication of the patient's hearing ability.

TUNING FORK TESTS

These are quick and simple to do: they require only a minimum of inexpensive equipment and give reliable, easily reproducible results. The most valuable tuning fork is one which vibrates at a rate of 512 cycles per second (512 hertz or Hz).

The prongs of the tuning fork are struck lightly on a firm (not hard) surface such as the examiner's knee or elbow, and then held next to the patient's ear. The patient is asked whether or not he hears the noise. With the vibrating fork held next to the ear canal in this way, the patient hears the sound by *air conduction*.

The flat base of the fork is then placed firmly on the mastoid bone behind the ear, and the patient is asked if he hears the sound. If he hears it he is asked whether it is louder or softer than the first sound. Sound heard in this way with the base of the fork on the mastoid bone is heard by *bone conduction*. The sound waves are conducted through the bones of the skull direct to the cochlear fluids.

In a normally functioning ear, sound is heard better by air conduction than by bone conduction due to the amplifying effect of the middle ear mechanism. This is called a *positive Rinne* response.

In cases of conductive deafness, sound transmitted by bone conduction will be heard better than by air conduction. This is known as a *negative Rinne* response.

In cases of sensori-neural deafness where the middle ear mechanism is functioning properly but the cochlea or the auditory nerve are defective, sound will still be heard better by air conduction than by bone conduction, so the *Rinne* will be *positive*.

There is one catch. If an ear is completely dead, a tuning fork held on the mastoid may be heard in the opposite ear and it will seem that *bone* conduction is better than air conduction. This is known as a *false negative Rinne*.

To summarise: (AC = air conduction; BC = bone conduction)

AC > BC	positive Rinne and is found in normal hearing and perceptive deafness
BC > AC	negative Rinne and is found in conductive deafness
BC > AC	with a 'dead' ear this finding is known as a false negative Rinne

WEBER TEST (Fig. 5/2)

A tuning fork is struck and placed in the centre of the forehead at an equal distance from each ear. The patient is asked in which ear he hears the sound louder.

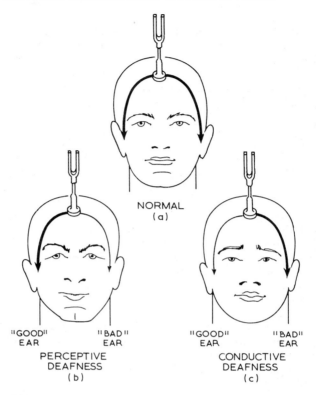

NORMAL
(a)

"GOOD"   "BAD"
EAR   EAR
PERCEPTIVE
DEAFNESS
(b)

"GOOD"   "BAD"
EAR   EAR
CONDUCTIVE
DEAFNESS
(c)

Fig. 5/2 The Weber test

In cases of unilateral perceptive deafness the sound will be heard in the ear with better hearing, i.e. the Weber is referred to the better hearing ear (Fig. 5/2b).

In cases of unilateral conductive hearing loss, the sound will be heard louder in the affected ear, i.e. the Weber will be referred to the apparently deafer ear (Fig. 5/2c).

PURE TONE AUDIOMETRY

An audiometer is a machine which is capable of producing pure tones electronically. These sounds can be made to vary in pitch (tone) and in loudness (intensity) and the machine is carefully calibrated (i.e. adjusted) so that the exact intensity of the tone is known accurately.

The test should be carried out in surroundings which are as free from unwanted noise as possible, preferably in a specially sound-proofed room.

To measure the threshold of hearing for air conduction the patient wears a pair of headphones connected to the machine and each ear is tested separately. At each test frequency the intensity of the sound is altered in small steps until the patient indicates the quietest possible sound that he can hear. This is the patient's threshold of hearing at this intensity and the process is repeated for all the test frequencies, and the points are indicated on a chart designed for the purpose. This represents the level of hearing for air conduction (Fig. 5/3a).

The threshold of hearing for bone conduction may then be measured for both ears but instead of using headphones, a small bone conduction transmitter is held firmly against the mastoid process by a spring headband. The results are then plotted on the same chart but using different symbols (Fig. 5/3b).

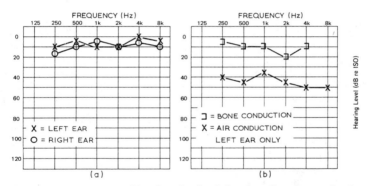

Fig. 5/3 Audiograms. (a) Showing level of hearing for air conduction (b) Showing level of hearing for bone conduction, and air conduction, e.g. otosclerosis

Masking

When there is a hearing loss in one ear only or when the hearing thresholds in the two ears are very different, care must be taken that the sounds meant for the poor ear are not being picked up in the better ear. When testing the hearing by air conduction with head-phones, a sound of 50 decibels will be transmitted across the skull and heard in the good ear. However, when testing bone conduction a sound of only 10 decibels will be transmitted through the bones of the skull to the better ear.

To overcome this phenomenon, the good ear must be kept occupied while the worse ear is tested. To do this the technique of *masking* is used. Masking noise (the sound made by an untuned television set (white noise) is found to be particularly useful) is played through one earphone to the good ear.

Interpretation of results

Once the hearing thresholds for air and bone conduction have been plotted on the charts, it can be seen if there is a difference between the two hearing levels (see Fig. 5/3b). If there is an *air-bone gap* this means that there is a conductive hearing loss in that ear. If the hearing loss is sensori-neural then the two curves are the same.

IMPEDANCE AUDIOMETRY (TYMPANOMETRY)
(Fig. 5/4)

This is a simple method of acquiring more information about the middle ear mechanism and is particularly useful in children when it can tell whether or not there is fluid in the middle ear.

Many pathological conditions make the tympanic membrane and middle ear systems stiff. When this happens sound waves will not be able to pass through to the cochlea. The ear drum has a high imped-ance. The impedance audiometer enables the doctor to take several measurements of impedance as the ear drum is artificially stiffened. If there is little change in the impedance this means that the tym-panic membrane was probably stiff to start with.

By changing the pressure in the ear canal the ear drum can be artificially stiffened. A normal ear drum is least stiff when the pres-sure on each side of the drum is equal, in other words when the pressure in the middle ear is the same as the pressure in the external ear (atmospheric pressure). The impedance audiometer works by bouncing low frequency sound on to the ear drum. If the drum is stiff most of the sound will bounce back into the ear canal. If the drum is compliant (compliance is the opposite to impedance) most of the sound passes through to the cochlea, and only a small amount is reflected back into the ear canal. The meter compares the sound

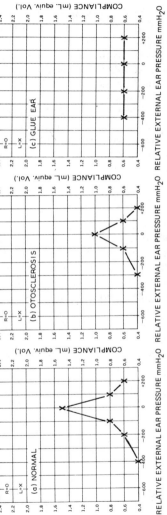

Fig. 5/4 Impedance audiometry. (a) Normal; (b) Otosclerosis; (c) Glue ear

level sent out with the sound level which bounces back into the ear canal. If the latter is high it suggests a stiff ear drum – high impedance.

The stiffness of an ear drum is measured in terms of its compliance. Normal ear drums are highly compliant unless they have been stiffened by some pathological process, or there is a marked difference between the pressure in the external ear and middle ear. Compliance is measured in millilitres equivalent (mlEquiv) ear volume, i.e. an ear which has a compliance of 2mlEquiv air volume has the same acoustic impedance as a hard-walled cavity of volume 2ml.

The change in compliance that occurs as the pressure in the external ear canal is changed by the impedance machine can then be plotted on a graph. In practice various different patterns are recognised and these give valuable information about the ear drum/middle ear system.

SPEECH AUDIOMETRY (Fig. 5/5)

While pure tone audiometry is a reliable method of testing hearing, one has to remember that it does no more than define the patient's ability to hear artificially produced sounds which have little relevance with regard to the patient's ability to hear the spoken word.

With speech audiometry, by using headphones and testing one ear at a time, the patient listens to a list of words, usually played on a tape recorder at a known sound intensity and has to repeat each word as he or she hears it. The tester scores each word right or wrong and a percentage 'score' is calculated for this intensity. Different word lists are played at different intensities, and the scores are plotted on a chart.

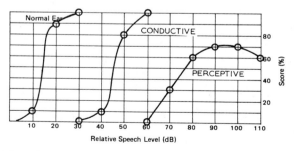

Fig. 5/5 Speech audiometry

Pure tone audiometry and speech audiometry depend on the patient's co-operation and concentration if the results are to be consistent. They are therefore *subjective* tests of hearing.

For patients who are unwilling or unable to co-operate to give reliable results, *objective* tests are used. The impedance audiogram is such a test. These tests do actually require the patients' co-operation inasmuch as they are required to sit still wearing a pair of headphones and not to fidget or fiddle with the equipment.

ELECTRIC RESPONSE AUDIOMETRY

These objective hearing tests give further valuable information particularly with respect to inner ear hearing loss.

All the nerve cells within the central nervous system produce tiny amounts of electrical activity when stimulated by the appropriate stimulus. This electrical activity can be recorded and measured on special machines, for example 'brain-waves' are recorded on an electro-encephalogram (EEG). The same is true of the ear.

If the ear is stimulated by sound, the hair cells within the cochlea will produce a minute amount of electrical activity and this will then be transmitted along the auditory nerve to the brainstem and so on through the various relay stations until the part of the cerebral cortex responsible for the reception of hearing is reached.

In order to pick up these tiny electrical impulses and to analyse them, sensitive recording electrodes are used. In the case of *electro-cochleography* (Fig. 5/6(a) and (b)) a tiny needle electrode is placed through the tympanic membrane, while for the examination known as *brainstem audiometry* the recording electrode is placed behind the ear on the skin of the mastoid process.

It has already been said that these amounts of electrical activity are small and they have to be distinguished from all the 'background' electrical activity going on in the rest of the brain. A computer is therefore used to carry out the analysis, and the results are displayed on an oscilloscope screen where they may either be photographed or recorded on special paper for future reference (Fig. 5/7). By altering the intensity of the sound presented to the ear, the threshold of hearing may be estimated.

This electrical activity arising from the ear is not affected by anaesthesia so this method of testing is particularly valuable in assessing the hearing level of certain babies or very young children who would otherwise not co-operate with hearing tests, e.g. due to

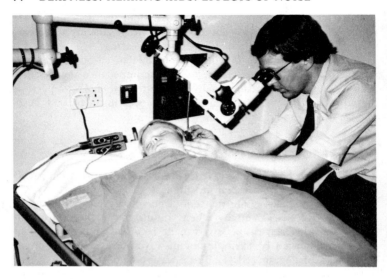

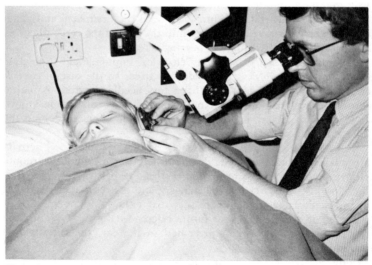

Fig. 5/6 a and b Electrocochleography. Inserting the electrode

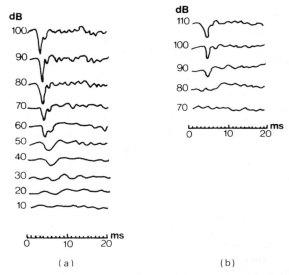

(a)   (b)

Fig. 5/7 A recording trace of an electrocochleogram. (a) A patient with normal hearing. The action potential can be traced down to 20dB; (b) A patient with impaired hearing. The action potential cannot be traced below 80dB

severe mental or physical handicap or emotional disturbance, and about whom there is some real concern regarding their ability to hear.

By looking at the exact shape of the recording obtained, tests of this type can also give valuable information on the exact site of a lesion causing a sensori-neural hearing loss and are sometimes of great help in the detection of an acoustic neuroma.

Because the test does not rely primarily on the co-operation of the patient to give an accurate result, tests of this type will give an accurate indication of the level of hearing in a patient who may be feigning deafness for one reason or another.

HEARING AIDS

A hearing aid is an aid to hearing. It cannot restore normal hearing but for many hearing-handicapped people it offers a means of overcoming some of the worst aspects of their disability.

Simply giving a deaf person a hearing aid is not enough. The degree of benefit which any deaf person may expect from an aid will depend on the type and the severity of the hearing loss but in all cases the patient will need time to adjust to the aid and to learn to hear and listen again. People who regularly come into contact with hearing-aid users are advised to speak slowly and clearly to them.

Basically most hearing aids are the same and consist of a microphone which picks up the sound, an amplifier to make the sound louder and an earphone which delivers the sound to the ear. Modern technology allows the amplified sound to be modified in different ways to compensate for different types of deafness.

Body-worn hearing aids have the earphones connected to the main part of the aid by a flexible wire (Fig. 5/8).

Behind-the-ear aids (Fig. 5/9) have the microphone within the case of the aid and the sound is delivered to the ear through a rigid curved plastic tube to which the ear-mould is connected by a short piece of flexible tubing.

The hearing aid is powered by batteries and it is important that the *right* batteries are fitted *correctly*.

Ear-moulds are individually made for each patient and should be a snug comfortable fit. If the mould is unsatisfactory or incorrectly fitted into the ear the aid will whistle when it is turned on. If the patient's hearing aid is making a whistling noise (feedback), check the ear-mould first to see that it is fitted correctly and then check that the volume control is not turned up too high.

Some patients with a very severe conductive hearing loss or chronically discharging ear or who are unable to wear an ear-mould, for example following a recent ear operation, may be helped by a bone conduction aid. Instead of the amplified sound being delivered through the ear-mould into the ear, sound reaches the patient via a small bone conductor held on to the mastoid process by a metal spring band.

Deaf patients in a ward can easily feel isolated and even ignored by other patients if there are difficulties with communication. It is vital that nurses and doctors are able to communicate with patients who are hard of hearing, so if any patient comes into hospital with a hearing aid it is important that the aid should be worn and that it should be working properly.

Nurses on an ENT ward should be able to recognise and deal with the more simple hearing-aid problems.

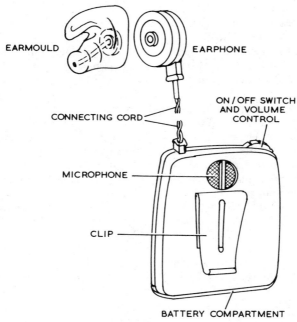

Fig. 5/8 A body-worn hearing aid

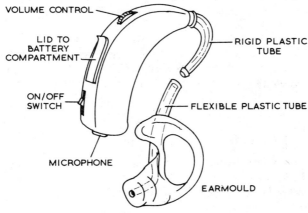

Fig. 5/9 A behind-the-ear hearing aid

Useful tips

If the sound is fading out, replace the batteries.

If there is no sound at all:

1. Check that the aid is switched on and the volume is turned up.
2. Replace battery and check that it is inserted the right way round.
3. Check that the ear-mould is not blocked with wax – if it is, clean it.
4. On body-worn aids, replace the cord (wire).
5. On behind-the-ear aids look at the flexible tube and if it is distorted or collapsed it will need replacing. Condensation may collect in the tube and may lead to blockage: if this happens remove the ear-mould and plastic tube and blow through it. Condensation in the rigid plastic tube can be removed by gently tapping with a finger but never blow directly into the aid.

If the sound gradually, or suddenly, becomes fainter, check the aid as above and if everything seems satisfactory tell the doctor. It may simply be that the ear is blocked by wax.

If the ear is sore inform the doctor.

If the aid is still not working then the problem should be referred to the hearing department. A faulty aid should be repaired or replaced.

Other aids for hearing

There are various other devices available to help deaf people at home and if the ward regularly has hearing-impaired patients they should know about the aids, for they can make the patients' stay in hospital more enjoyable. Patients should also be told of what aids can be obtained for use in their own homes. Such aids include amplified telephones, earphones for use with the radio or television and a loop system to enable hearing-aid users to listen to television more clearly.

Lip-reading

For severely deaf patients, or patients with steadily worsening deafness, lip-reading classes should be considered. A member of the hearing-aid department or the local hearing therapist will be able to give advice.

THE EFFECTS OF NOISE ON THE EAR

For many years it has been recognised that loud noise can damage hearing. The effects of prolonged exposure to loud noise, whether industrial, e.g. sheet metal working, sporting, e.g. due to firing a shot gun, or due to loud music in discos, are the same. Initially the deafness and associated tinnitus may be *temporary* and the hearing quickly returns to normal after a period of quiet, away from the source of the noise. After prolonged exposure, however, the hearing loss becomes *permanent* and may be accompanied by high pitched tinnitus.

Figure 5/10a is a typical audiogram and shows a loss of hearing at 4000 Hz. This frequency is higher than the normal range of speech frequencies (250–2000 Hz) so the patient may be unaffected by this deafness in normal conversation, but as the deafness progresses (Fig. 5/10b) the degree of deafness worsens and comes to involve the speech frequencies. At this point the patient will begin to notice increasingly severe difficulties with hearing and the tinnitus will become more troublesome.

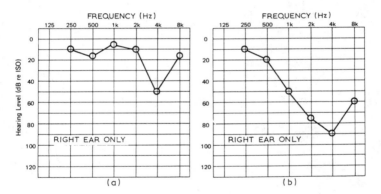

Fig. 5/10 (a) and (b) Audiogram of noise-induced hearing loss to show progression of deafness

Once the noise-induced hearing loss is established there is no cure, so it is important to take all possible precautions to eliminate exposure to noise and to recognise any deafness early.

Prevention

At work the source of noise may be suppressed, by modifying the design of machinery, or by sound-proofing noisy parts of a machine. In parts of a factory where noise is recognised as being above the desired level, warning notices must be displayed and personnel must wear protection (ear plugs or ear defenders) and they should not be exposed to high levels of noise for any longer than absolutely necessary. Noisy places of work should be identified and the noise levels carefully measured using special equipment. Personnel exposed to noise should have a hearing test before taking up employment and at regular intervals thereafter.

Noise-induced hearing loss is a recognised industrial disease for which compensation may be payable. Noise-induced hearing loss due to non-industrial causes such as noisy sports or hobbies is no less severe and demands the same precautions to prevent exposure and permanent damage to hearing.

FURTHER READING

Code of Practice for Reducing the Exposure of Employed Persons to Noise. HMSO, London.

CHAPTER SIX

Earache

Pain in the ear is usually due to inflammation which may be in the middle ear – otitis media – or external ear – otitis externa. The otitis externa may be diffuse or it may be localised in the form of a furuncle (a boil).

A common cause of earache, especially in children, is due to Eustachian tube dysfunction. As the Eustachian tube becomes blocked, the air within the middle ear cavity becomes absorbed through the mucous membrane and the tympanic membrane becomes indrawn. This stretching of the ear drum is painful and may cause the child to wake at night with earache.

There are other causes of earache which are not the result of diseases within the ear: these include diseases of the teeth, tongue, tonsils, pharynx, larynx, nose, sinuses, nasopharynx, temporomandibular joint and cervical spine, all of which may give rise to pain which is *referred* to the ear.

Therefore all these structures should be examined when a patient complains of earache and examifiation of the ear itself shows no abnormality.

OTITIS MEDIA

Acute otitis media describes the acute inflammation of the whole of the lining of the middle ear cleft. It is a common illness affecting predominantly young children.

From the time of birth, whenever a child swallows, air travels up the Eustachian tube into the middle ear cavity and equalises the pressure on each side of the tympanic membrane. Provided the pressure within the middle ear remains atmospheric, the air cell system within the mastoid will continue to develop outwards from the mastoid antrum. *Pneumatisation* is the name given to the process by which the system of air cells develops in the mastoid bone (Fig. 6/1). This process of pneumatisation continues until the age of about 12 years.

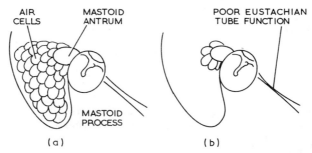

Fig. 6/1 Pneumatisation. (a) Well pneumatised; (b) Poorly pneumatised

Causes of acute otitis media (Fig. 6/2)

1. Following infectious diseases of the nose or nasopharynx, e.g. the common cold.
2. A large pad of infected adenoids may block the Eustachian tube. The air in the middle ear becomes absorbed and replaced by mucus which then becomes infected.
3. Muco-pus from infected sinuses may spread into the nasopharynx and infect the Eustachian tubes.
4. Through a perforation in the tympanic membrane.

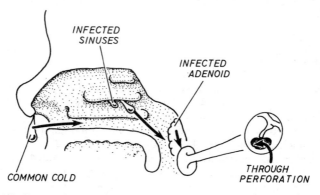

Fig. 6/2 Causes of acute otitis media

Pathology
The whole of the mucous membrane lining the middle ear cleft becomes acutely inflamed and produces muco-pus. The tympanic membrane also becomes inflamed and reddened, and as the amount of muco-pus increases, the pressure within the middle ear rises. The tympanic membrane stretches and eventually ruptures due to ischaemic necrosis. Muco-pus then discharges through the perforation into the ear canal. As the infection subsides with appropriate treatment, the perforation heals and the Eustachian tube functions once more.

Symptoms and signs
The symptoms of acute otitis media are earache, deafness, malaise and fever, followed by ear discharge.

The child may be generally unwell with a fever, vomiting and diarrhoea. If the temperature rises very high, the child may have a fit.

Severe earache may cause the child to cry and to wake at night. This pain is usually relieved when the ear discharges.

The tympanic membrane gradually becomes more red until it bulges and eventually ruptures. The discharge, containing a small amount of blood, may fill the external canal and pulsate. A light shone into the ear will reflect on the pulsating discharge: the 'light-house sign'.

The mastoid process is examined for swelling and tenderness. If the disease is treated efficiently in the early stages, it may be prevented from progressing to complications, the drum will heal and the hearing will return to its former level.

Treatment
The child should be put to bed, given plenty of fluids to drink and analgesics such as aspirin or paracetamol prescribed. Decongestant mixtures by mouth may relieve mucosal congestion in the nose and Eustachian tube. Once the clinical diagnosis has been made antibiotics may be prescribed and should be continued for seven days. If the antibiotics are not taken for the full duration of the course, the infection may not be fully eradicated and may recur quickly.

Complications (Fig. 6/3)

FAILURE TO RESOLVE
If the antibiotics have not been taken for long enough or if the
bacteria are resistant to the particular antibiotic chosen, the infecting
organism may remain in the middle ear.

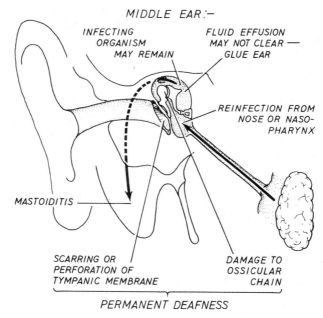

Fig. 6/3 Complication of acute otitis media

RECURRENCE
If the infection appears to resolve completely but then recurs rapidly,
the most likely cause is a focus of infection elsewhere in the upper
respiratory tract, such as infected adenoids or sinuses. These two
conditions may have to be dealt with surgically.

DEAFNESS
Once the infection has subsided mucus may remain in the middle
ear and may be removed by a *myringotomy*, perhaps with insertion
of a *grommet* (see p. 67).

Repeated attacks of otitis media may cause scarring of the tympanic membrane or damage to the ossicular chain possibly resulting in permanent deafness.

Acute mastoiditis
If acute otitis media is left untreated or is treated inadequately, the infection of the mucous membrane may spread to involve the bony partitions between the air cells in the mastoid. The bony partitions break down with discharge of muco-pus from the ear. There is a red tender swelling behind the ear which pushes the pinna forward and downward.

This condition is really an abscess in the mastoid bone and the treatment is surgical, namely drainage. The mastoid is opened through a skin incision behind the ear and the infected air cells are drained by removing the bony cell walls along with the infected contents. This is known as *cortical mastoidectomy* (see p. 71).

Acute mastoiditis is now far less common in the United Kingdom because antibiotics are given more readily for otitis media but the condition is still seen from time to time, often in young children.

CHRONIC SUPPURATIVE OTITIS MEDIA (CSOM)
(Fig. 6/4)

This is a long-standing condition in which the ear discharges. There are two varieties: *safe* CSOM (tubo-tympanic disease) and *unsafe* CSOM (attico-antral disease). There are definite differences between

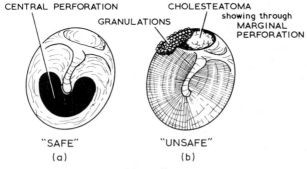

Fig. 6/4 Chronic suppurative otitis media

the two types and the distinction between them is of considerable practical importance.

Safe (tubo-tympanic) CSOM (Fig. 6/4a)

As a result of frequent middle ear infections there is a perforation in the central part of the tympanic membrane – the pars tensa. There may also be damage to the ossicles, particularly to the long process of the incus because this slender piece of bone has a precarious blood supply.

This type of otitis media is often associated with disease elsewhere in the upper respiratory tract; this should be sought and treated as well. Serious complications do not occur.

Patients should be urged to keep the ear clean and dry. Waterproof ear plugs, made by impregnating cotton wool with petroleum jelly, worn when swimming, bathing or washing the hair will prevent water entering the ear.

The perforation in the tympanic membrane may be closed by the operation of *myringoplasty* (see p. 68).

Deafness is of the conductive type and although the operation of myringoplasty and ossiculoplasty may be performed to improve the hearing, the residual deafness may require a hearing aid.

Unsafe (attico-antral) CSOM (Fig. 6/4b)

In these cases the perforation occurs at the margin of the tympanic membrane either posteriorly or superiorly in the attic region. The tympanic membrane first becomes retracted as the result of long-standing negative pressure in the middle ear and in this retraction pocket a *cholesteatoma* develops.

CHOLESTEATOMA

This is the name given to a collection of keratinising squamous epithelium within the middle ear. It occurs in ears where the mastoid bone has failed to become filled with air cells (i.e. poorly pneumatised) because of poor Eustachian tube function.

Air is absorbed from the middle ear cleft more quickly than it can be replaced via the malfunctioning Eustachian tube. This means that for much of the time there is a negative pressure in the middle ear. Thus the ear drum tends to be drawn inward. The weakest part of the drum, and therefore the part most likely to become indrawn, is the pars flaccida. This is likely to result in a small pocket being formed in the attic region. This pocket becomes filled with squamous epithelial cells which are constantly being produced by the epithelial layer on the surface of the tympanic membrane. This collection of dead skin cells is now known as a *cholesteatoma* and gradually enlarges. As it enlarges, it erodes any bone with which it comes into contact by a combination of pressure necrosis and enzymic digestion. The outer attic wall becomes eroded and if the cholesteatoma becomes infected the ear will begin to discharge foul-smelling pus through the perforation. Erosion of the ossicles will give rise to deafness.

This aggressive type of disease is particularly likely to result in complications if left untreated and therefore fully merits the name of unsafe otitis media.

A patient with a cholesteatoma should attend the ENT clinic for regular thorough aural toilet. The ear is dry mopped with cotton wool and all the epithelial debris removed. This is best done by suction using the operating microscope. Provided the ear remains clean and dry, the hearing remains stable, and all the squamous epithelium can be removed, then the ear may simply be kept under observation. If the discharge continues, the deafness increases, or if the patient develops any of the complications of chronic suppurative otitis media, then a radical mastoidectomy must be performed.

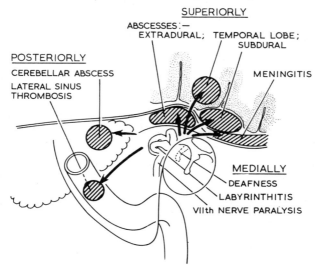

Fig. 6/5 Complications arising from a cholesteatoma

MANAGEMENT OF THE DISEASE (see p. 73)

COMPLICATIONS (Fig. 6/5)
If you remember the anatomy of the ear and the structures situated near by, it is comparatively simple to define the possible complications.

1. If the cholesteatoma erodes *backwards* (posteriorly), lateral venous sinus thrombosis and cerebellar abscess may occur.

2. If the cholesteatoma erodes *superiorly*, the following may occur: extradural abscess, meningitis, subdural abscess or temporal lobe abscess.

3. If the cholesteatoma erodes *medially*, the following may occur:
   (a) *Labyrinthitis* with severe vertigo as the lateral semicircular canal is eroded.
   (b) VIIth cranial (facial) nerve paralysis.
   (c) *Deafness:* damage to the ossicular chain will result in conductive deafness but the hearing loss may become total and sensori-neural as the cochlea is eroded.

CHAPTER SEVEN

Nursing Management for Ear Surgery

COMMUNICATION

Patients who are admitted for ear operations generally have one problem in common – they almost all suffer from some degree of deafness. It is therefore essential that the nurse realises the potential difficulties in communication and takes steps to make things as easy as possible for the patient. During conversation the nurse should stand in front of the patient preferably with a light shining on the nurse's face so that the patient can see her face and particularly her lips more easily. If the nurse stands with her back to a bright window the patient will have increased and unnecessary difficulty. The nurse should speak clearly and slowly and if the patient does not seem to understand she must not be tempted to shout for this will not help; it is better to try re-phrasing the statement or question and to use different words which the patient may find easier to lip read.

There are numerous mechanical aids available to assist the hard of hearing on an ENT ward; indeed they would be helpful on any ward which caters for the elderly, many of whom may be deaf. Such aids include telephones with amplifiers, and loop systems to enable hearing-aid wearers to listen to TV more easily. It is also sensible to have a stock of hearing-aid batteries or to have access to spare hearing aids as a temporary measure. Even the old fashioned ear trumpet, though cumbersome, can provide excellent benefit to some very deaf patients.

Immediately a patient is admitted to the ward the nursing process should be implemented (see Chapter 2). With all patients requiring routine surgery the care plan can be divided into pre- and post-operative requirements.

PRE-OPERATIVE CARE

Apart from the general notes which will be entered on the care plan and are relevant to all surgical cases – e.g. consent, no food and drink before surgery, premedication – the following points should be particularly recorded.

1. Explanation

The details of the operation will be explained to the patient or, in the case of a child, to the parents, by a doctor. The patient may well ask the nurse questions and one of the more senior nurses on the ward should take the opportunity of explaining about the operation with particular reference to factors which will be of relevance to the nursing management postoperatively. As indicated previously it greatly helps if the nurse can be present when the doctor explains any surgery to the patient. Specific details which the nurse may wish to discuss with the patient include:

(a) Ear dressings. The ear canal may well contain a dressing after the operation and this may therefore make the patient seem more deaf. Following some operations, e.g. mastoidectomy, the ear will be dressed with a mastoid bandage.

(b) Length of stay in hospital. This will obviously depend on post-operative progress but the patient will find it helpful to know roughly how long he will be in hospital.

2. Facial nerve (VIIth cranial)

The facial nerve which controls the movement of the facial muscles runs through the ear and is therefore at risk from disease of the ears or from ear surgery (see p. 29). The nurse must particularly note the symmetry of facial movements and if there is any abnormality of facial movements prior to operation it should be carefully noted in the nursing assessment.

3. Audiogram

The patient should have an up-to-date audiogram pre-operatively (see p. 39). Special mastoid radiographs may need to be arranged together with any investigations, e.g. full blood count (FBC) and a chest radiograph.

4. Shave

For certain operations, e.g. mastoidectomy or myringoplasty, some surgeons ask for an aural shave, i.e. the removal of the hair within 2cm of the pinna. Before doing this the nurse must check in the notes which ear is going to be operated upon. No shave is required for a stapedectomy.

5. Antibiotic cover
This may be prescribed by the surgeon for patients undergoing stapedectomy. In such cases it must be clearly recorded on the care plan.

POSTOPERATIVE CARE

The following points should be carefully recorded on the care plan:

1. Airway
Following all operations it is vital to ensure that the patient has a clear air way and is breathing freely. If there is a recovery ward, the patient may be kept there until he is fully conscious before returning to the ward.

2. Position
The patient should be lying comfortably with the head on a pillow and with the operated ear uppermost for 12 hours.

3. Facial movements
At admission the nurse will have noted whether there were signs of asymmetry and will have recorded this fact accordingly. After surgery the nurse must carefully observe facial movements for any sign of asymmetry which might have resulted from the surgery. If there is an abnormality, or if there is any doubt, the doctor should be informed at once.

4. Temperature: pulse: respiration
The temperature, pulse and respiration will be monitored regularly.

5. Anti-emetics and sedation
After some major ear operations the patient is liable to feel giddy and sick. The nurse may be able to observe rhythmical eye movements (nystagmus). The patient's discomfort will be eased by an anti-emetic drug such as prochlorperazine given intramuscularly or by suppository. Most ear operations are not particularly painful so

the patient is unlikely to require much in the way of analgesia; however, sedation is important following a stapedectomy to prevent the patient from moving about too much and possibly dislodging the piston.

6. Change of dressing

If a mastoid bandage has been applied in theatre it is usually advisable to remove it and re-apply it after 24 hours. Cotton wool in the meatus should be changed, with care being taken not to remove any dressings which are in the ear canal itself. At the same time any wound drains can be inspected and removed if drainage has ceased.

After two or three days the mastoid bandage may be removed and the ear covered by a dry dressing. For children it is better to keep the mastoid bandage on for longer to keep little fingers out of the wound.

Any packing in the ear canal is left until it is removed by the doctor; the length of time it stays in will depend on the type of operation as well as the personal preference of the surgeon. The first dressing may be changed in theatre under a short anaesthetic but thereafter it can usually be done on the ward or in the outpatient's department by a doctor or a trained nurse.

7. Sutures

These are usually removed after seven days.

PROCEDURES WHICH A NURSE MAY PERFORM

Ear drops

Instilling ear drops is a very simple procedure.

EQUIPMENT
A tray with:
   (a) the ear drops to be given
   (b) sterile cotton wool balls.

METHOD
The nurse washes her hands and asks the patient to lie on his side, with his head on a pillow, with the ear to be treated uppermost. With one hand the nurse should hold the pinna and gently pull upwards and slightly backward so as to straighten the ear canal. The

drops are then inserted into the canal and a piece of cotton wool put into the entrance of the ear canal. The patient is asked to remain on his side for about five minutes so that the drops can be absorbed.

Ear syringing

This should only be done on instructions from the doctor and *never* if there is any possibility of a perforated ear drum.

Before attempting to syringe wax out of the ears, drops, such as warmed olive oil, should have been inserted into the ear canal at least over the previous 24 hours so as to soften the wax.

EQUIPMENT
1. Metal ear syringe with detachable nozzle
2. Auriscope and speculum
3. Lotion to be used, warmed to a temperature of 37°C
4. Receiver, e.g. kidney dish
5. Mackintosh cape
6. Towel
7. Cotton wool balls
8. Aural forceps
9. Two bags – one for soiled swabs and one for soiled instruments

METHOD

Good lighting is essential if the procedure is to be carried out thoroughly and safely. This is best achieved if the nurse wears a head mirror to reflect light from a bull's-eye lamp, or similar, on to the patient's ear.

The patient should sit with the ear to be syringed towards the nurse. A mackintosh cape is placed around the patient's shoulders with a towel on top. The patient is asked to hold the kidney dish close against the cheek under the ear. The nurse, having washed and dried her hands, attaches the nozzle to the syringe and fills it with the warmed solution, e.g. normal saline. The air is expelled from the syringe and the tip of the nozzle is inserted in the entrance of the ear canal. With her other hand the nurse holds the pinna and gently pulls it upward and slightly backward to straighten the canal. The solution is expelled towards the roof of the canal so that it is forced over the debris or wax and forced back along the floor, washing the wax out with it.

The patient should tip his head on to that side to let any excess water drain out and then the ear should be dried with cotton wool.

The nurse should check with the auriscope that there is no wax or debris left and that the canal is dry. If there are still signs of wax or debris the canal could be gently cleaned with a piece of cotton wool using aural forceps.

The equipment should be cleared away and the nozzle of the syringe washed and sterilised before re-use.

Before the patient is discharged the nurse should make sure that the patient is not dizzy. Dizziness may result if the solution is not at body temperature. Any dizziness should last only for a minute or two.

Specific nursing points relating to various surgical procedures will be indicated in the relevant section in Chapter 8.

CHAPTER EIGHT

Surgical Procedures

The majority of procedures considered in this chapter involve the middle ear structures, namely the tympanic membrane and ossicles, and the mastoid air cell system.

SURGICAL APPROACHES TO THE EAR

The three main ways of access to the middle ear are permeatal, endaural and postaural. The choice is governed by the actual operation and by the structures that the surgeon particularly wishes to view.

Permeatal

This means going down the external auditory meatus itself. It is a suitable approach for myringotomy and for insertion of a grommet, stapedectomy, and some forms of myringoplasty.

Endaural (Fig. 8/1a)

An incision is made just in front of the pinna and is then extended downward into the ear canal. It allows the opening of the external auditory canal to be opened more widely so that a better view may be obtained of the deeper parts of the canal and tympanic membrane.

It is a suitable approach for the removal of small tumours of the ear canal and for repairing perforations of the tympanic membrane.

By extending the incision slightly, and further freeing the pinna, the mastoid bone may be exposed allowing mastoid operations to be performed.

Postaural (Fig. 8/1b)

An incision is made in the skin behind the ear, and the ear pulled forward. This provides immediate access to the mastoid bone. Myringoplasty may also be done by this route.

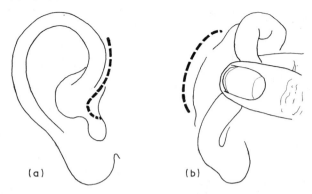

Fig. 8/1 Surgical approaches to the ear. (a) Endaural; (b) Postaural

Nursing note

If either an endaural or a postaural approach is anticipated, or a separate skin incision is going to be made, for example, to obtain a piece of temporalis fascia for repair of a tympanic membrane perforation, then the skin around the pinna should be carefully and thoroughly shaved for a distance of 2cm. The shaving should be done on the ward before the premedication is given. This enables the skin to be cleaned more thoroughly in theatre and will stop hair getting into the wound and introducing infection.

MYRINGOTOMY (Fig. 8/2)

This is the name given to an incision made in the tympanic membrane. It is usually done to remove fluid from the middle ear or to insert a grommet.

The fluid may be infected in acute suppurative otitis media which either has been untreated or has failed to respond to the treatment with antibiotics. The need to release this pus from the middle ear occurs far less frequently nowadays due to the more widespread use of antibiotics. The procedure is, however, a satisfying one as far as the patient is concerned since he will be relieved immediately of the intense, throbbing earache of acute suppurative otitis media.

A specimen of the pus may be sent to the laboratory for bacteriological investigation. In *serous otitis media* the fluid is invariably sterile.

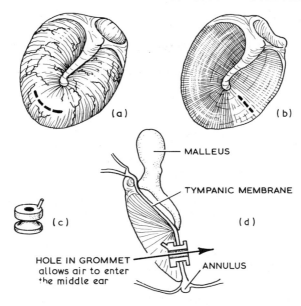

Fig. 8/2 Myringotomy. (a) Acute otitis media; (b) Glue ear; (c) A grommet; (d) Cross-section of the ear to show a grommet in position

For the latter conditions a *grommet* may be necessary. A grommet is a tiny tube, usually made of plastic, which may be inserted into the myringotomy incision (Fig. 8/2c). The main function of the grommet is to allow air to enter the middle ear space (this is the same function as the Eustachian tube (see p. 29)) but the tube may also allow some of the middle ear fluid to drain away.

The question may be asked, Why is the middle ear fluid present? The most important factor influencing the health of the middle ear is the Eustachian tube. If this fails to open properly and does not allow air at atmospheric pressure to pass from the nasopharynx into the middle ear, then the middle ear will not function as it should and the cause of Eustachian tube dysfunction should be sought.

In *children* it is commonly believed that the presence of enlarged adenoids contributes towards the formation of a middle ear effusion. Adenoidectomy is therefore performed at the same time as insertion of a grommet. Any disease which might be evident in the upper respiratory tract should be dealt with at the same time, for example chronically infected tonsils may be removed or a maxillary sinusitis drained.

In the *adult* the same rules apply and a middle ear effusion must be regarded as a sign of disease elsewhere in the nose or nasopharynx. In particular, the post-nasal space should be carefully examined to exclude the presence of a carcinoma blocking the opening of the Eustachian tube.

Nursing points

Following the insertion of a grommet the nurse must explain to the patient (if an adult) or to the parents (if a child) that water must be kept out of the ear. Waterproof ear plugs (cotton wool impregnated with petroleum jelly) should be worn in the bath or when washing the hair. Swimming is not allowed. If water is allowed to get into the ear canal it may go through the hole in the grommet and may give rise to an ear infection.

MYRINGOPLASTY (Fig. 8/3)

This is the operation to repair a perforation of the tympanic membrane. A perforation may follow infection or trauma. Reasons for wanting to repair a perforated ear drum are:

1. If the patient wishes to go swimming.
2. If the patient wishes to join the Armed Forces.
3. To improve the hearing.

The material usually used to repair the perforation is temporalis fascia. This is the tough, fibrous covering of the temporalis muscle which lies on the side of the skull, above the ear. The fascia is strong and easy to use and has the advantage of being readily available from the patient himself.

The operation may be performed permeatally, in which case a

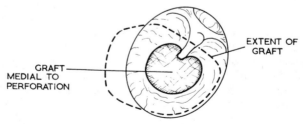

Fig. 8/3 Myringoplasty

separate incision must be made to obtain the temporalis fascia. Otherwise the operation is done via an endaural or postaural approach (see Fig. 8/1).

The 'patch' of temporalis fascia is usually placed underneath, i.e. medial to, the tympanic membrane and it will stick to the tympanic membrane remnant as a result of the surface tension of the blood.

The ear canal is lightly packed with a piece of ribbon gauze impregnated with an antiseptic material such as bismuth, iodoform and liquid paraffin (BIPP Gauze). If an incision has been made in the skin, this is sutured and a bandage applied to the ear for 24 hours. Some surgeons like antibiotics to be given to lessen the likelihood of the ears becoming infected.

Specific nursing points

General nursing management is discussed in Chapter 2. Specifically, following myringoplasty the nurse must ensure that the patient does *not* blow his nose for at least two weeks. The graft can become detached if the nose is blown forcefully causing air to be blown up the Eustachian tube into the middle ear.

The patient is usually in hospital for about five days, and his sutures may be taken out pre-discharge or left in to be removed subsequently by his family doctor. After myringoplasty the patient should be advised to take life easily at home for at least two weeks before returning to work.

OSSICULOPLASTY (Fig. 8/4)

Parts of one or more ossicles may be eroded by repeated attacks of otitis media. The most common defect is for the long process of the incus to be missing, though the crura of the stapes may also be absent. More rarely the ossicles may be fractured or displaced as a result of trauma, for example a blow on the head.

Such a defect in the ossicular chain will give rise to a conductive deafness and if the deafness is to be corrected, then the continuity of the ossicular chain must be restored by an operation. Such an operation is termed an *ossiculoplasty*.

Many tiny ingenious prostheses have been designed. The initial prostheses were made of plastic but were quickly rejected and extruded from the ear. Pieces of nasal septal cartilage shaped and reinforced with fine stainless steel wire were then used but were not very rigid and often became dislodged.

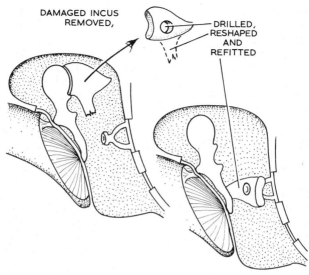

Fig. 8/4 Ossiculoplasty

The next development came when it was recognised that ossicles removed from cadavers and preserved in alcohol could be placed in the middle ear without being rejected. The preserved ossicles, known as homografts, could be drilled to fit exactly the requirements of the ear being operated on. These ossicles which are essentially dead bone become revitalised by new bone growing into them along the vascular channels of the dead bone.

If the patient's own incus is only partly damaged, it may be removed, reshaped and repositioned between the malleus and the incus to conduct sound waves once more.

TYMPANOPLASTY

In this operation all the active disease of the middle ear and mastoid is removed and the sound-conducting mechanism is reconstructed. It may consist of a myringoplasty or an ossiculoplasty, or both.

MEATOPLASTY

This is an operation to enlarge the opening of the external auditory meatus. It forms an essential part of any mastoidectomy operation to allow good access to the mastoid cavity for cleaning purposes.

MASTOIDECTOMY (Fig. 8/5)

Cortical mastoidectomy (Fig. 8/5a)

This is performed for acute mastoiditis following otitis media (see p. 55) or for secretory otitis media (glue ear).

Acute mastoiditis: This is a complication of otitis media in which there is a breakdown of the bony walls of the mastoid air cells. The condition occurs less commonly since the more widespread use of antibiotics to treat acute otitis media. The patient is usually a child who is ill with a raised temperature and a mucopurulent ear discharge. There is a tender swelling over the mastoid process and the overlying skin is inflamed. Acute mastoiditis is essentially an abscess occurring in the mastoid bone and, like all abscesses, it must be drained.

Recurrent glue ear: In some children secretory otitis media persists even after repeated myringotomy and aspiration, after adenoidectomy and elimination of any source of infection in the upper respiratory tract. In such children it is often of benefit to perform a cortical mastoidectomy to eliminate any focus of lingering inflammation or infection, or cholesterol granuloma in the mastoid.

OPERATION

The operation is usually performed via a postaural approach (Fig. 8/1b). The mastoid antrum is opened and all the diseased air cells are removed using a drill. Because this condition usually occurs in a mastoid with many air cells (well pneumatised) the resultant cavity may be quite large. The size of the cavity is limited in an upward direction by the middle fossa dura and posteriorly by the lateral venous sinus which drains blood from the brain. The bony wall between the mastoid and the middle ear and external auditory canal is retained.

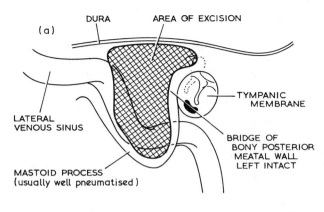

(a)

DURA

AREA OF EXCISION

TYMPANIC MEMBRANE

BRIDGE OF BONY POSTERIOR MEATAL WALL LEFT INTACT

LATERAL VENOUS SINUS

MASTOID PROCESS (usually well pneumatised)

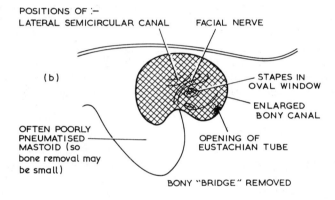

POSITIONS OF :–
LATERAL SEMICIRCULAR CANAL

FACIAL NERVE

(b)

STAPES IN OVAL WINDOW

ENLARGED BONY CANAL

OFTEN POORLY PNEUMATISED MASTOID (so bone removal may be small)

OPENING OF EUSTACHIAN TUBE

BONY "BRIDGE" REMOVED

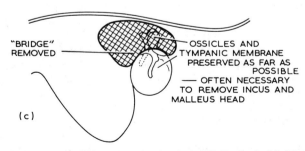

"BRIDGE" REMOVED

OSSICLES AND TYMPANIC MEMBRANE PRESERVED AS FAR AS POSSIBLE
— OFTEN NECESSARY TO REMOVE INCUS AND MALLEUS HEAD

(c)

Fig. 8/5 Types of mastoidectomy. (a) Cortical; (b) Radical; (c) Modified radical

The wound is sutured and a small drain is left in until any discharge ceases.

The perforation in the tympanic membrane will often close spontaneously once the infection has settled down but until it does, the ear canal should be kept clean and dry by gentle dry mopping (see p. 74).

Radical mastoidectomy (Fig. 8/5b)

This is performed for chronic suppurative otitis media (see p. 56). All the cholesteatoma is removed along with the diseased bone of the mastoid air cells. The tympanic membrane and ossicles which are already damaged by disease are removed leaving only the stapes to prevent damage to the inner ear. The bony wall between the middle ear and mastoid is then taken away to provide one big cavity. This last step is performed very carefully to avoid damage to the facial nerve as it crosses the middle ear.

The opening of the external auditory canal is then enlarged to provide easy access to the cavity for cleaning purposes.

After stitching the skin incision, the cavity is packed with BIPP Gauze (see p. 69). The wound is covered with a sterile gauze dressing and a mastoid bandage is applied.

NURSING NOTE
When the patient recovers from the anaesthetic it is very important for the nurse to look for movements of the facial muscles since lack of movement on one side may indicate damage to the facial nerve during the operation and the surgeon should be notified at once.

Modified radical mastoidectomy (Fig. 8/5c)

This is also performed for chronic suppurative otitis media but if the cholesteatoma is small it may be possible, after eradicating all of the cholesteatoma and diseased bone, to preserve part of the tympanic membrane and part of the malleus.

Preservation of part of the ossicular chain and part of the tympanic membrane may make it easier to reconstruct the sound-conducting mechanism. The cavity is often smaller and easier to manage postoperatively but otherwise the postoperative care is exactly the same as for a radical mastoidectomy.

AFTER-CARE OF THE MASTOID CAVITY
After one or two weeks the BIPP Gauze packing may be removed and the cavity dry mopped.

Dry mopping: This is done by a doctor or by an experienced nurse and it is usually convenient to carry out the procedure in the treatment room with the patient seated. Good lighting, e.g. using a bull's-eye lamp and a head mirror, is essential. After the nurse has washed her hands the ear to be mopped is inspected and any dressing in the ear canal is removed, using forceps which are then discarded. A small piece of cotton wool is securely attached to a suitable applicator such as a Jobson-Horne probe (see Fig. 1/1, p. 2) or a wooden orange stick, and the cotton wool is then put into the opening in the ear canal to mop up any moisture or debris. At all times the operator must remember that the ear is a sensitive structure and in the presence of inflammation it will be even more so. Gentleness is therefore vital. By gently pulling the pinna upward and backward the ear canal is straightened making mopping and subsequent inspection of the ear canal or cavity easier. Soiled cotton wool should be discarded and fresh cotton wool re-applied to the applicator. The procedure is repeated until the ear canal is as clean and dry as possible. If necessary, drops or powder may be instilled as prescribed or a small piece of sterile cotton wool placed in the entrance of the meatus. The cavity should be dry mopped at regular intervals once . or twice a week and any excess granulation tissue removed with a 10% solution of silver nitrate on a small cotton wool applicator. The cavity will eventually become dry and lined by skin. When this point is reached, the patient needs only to attend at intervals of 6 to 12 months for removal of wax and dead skin from the cavity.

If the cavity does not become completely dry, and some of them do not, then the patient may need to attend the outpatient department more regularly for cleaning. Alternatively, patients can be taught by the doctor or nurse how to gently dry mop their own ears using cotton wool on an orange stick. The tip of the stick must be well covered and the doctor or nurse should watch the patient doing it for one or two times.

STAPEDECTOMY (Fig. 8/6)

This is the operation of choice in the treatment of otosclerosis.

Otosclerosis: In this condition the footplate of the stapes bone is prevented from moving fully by the presence of tiny, abnormal outgrowths of bone around the oval window. Because the stapes cannot move, sound waves which strike the tympanic membrane are not

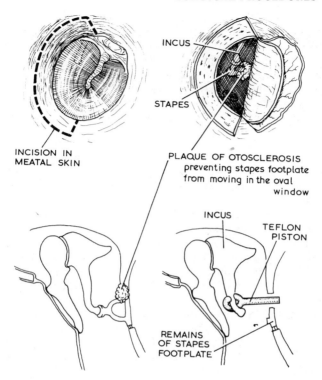

INCUS

STAPES

INCISION IN
MEATAL SKIN

PLAQUE OF OTOSCLEROSIS
preventing stapes footplate
from moving in the oval
window

INCUS

TEFLON
PISTON

REMAINS
OF STAPES
FOOTPLATE

Fig. 8/6 Stapedectomy

transmitted properly through the ossicles to the organ of hearing,
the cochlea. This means that the patient will be deaf (see Fig. 5/3,
p. 39).

The condition tends to affect women more than men, is usually
noticed in young adult life and may be present in one or both ears.
There is often a strong family history and, if the condition occurs in
a young woman, the deafness may become worse during pregnancy.

The operation
Using the operating microscope an incision is made around the margin of the tympanic membrane and the posterior half of the drum is

turned forward, like the page of a book. It is then possible to get a good view of the stapes sitting in the oval window and of the joint between the incus and stapes bones. The crura of the stapes and part of the stapes footplate are carefully removed and a piston, made usually of plastic or stainless steel, is attached to the incus. The other end of the piston reaches into the little hole in the stapes footplate so that sound waves may, once more, be transmitted via the ear drum and ossicles to the cochlea, and the patient's hearing restored. The ear drum is folded back to its original position and the operation is complete.

NURSING CARE

The patient is nursed on his side with the operated ear uppermost, to reduce to a minimum the possibility of the piston's falling out. General nursing management is discussed on page 61, but the following points are stressed:

1. Bed rest is necessary for the first 24 hours because any excessive movement may dislodge the piston. The patient is likely to feel nauseated and giddy and for this reason as well it would be dangerous to get out of bed unaided. The patient may be allowed to use a commode.
2. Regular anti-emetics will be required.
3. The patient has to be told not to blow his nose hard for six weeks in case the piston becomes dislodged.
4. The patient should be advised to avoid bending or to turn his head suddenly.
5. The length of stay in hospital is usually seven days.

Stapedectomy is probably the most fiddly of all operations on the ear, and it carries a substantial risk of damage to the inner ear with permanent and perhaps total deafness. This complication may occur not only at the time of operation but it has been reported as occurring more than 10 years later. For this reason it is advisable to operate on one ear only.

As an alternative to operation, patients with otosclerosis may be offered a hearing aid (see Chapter 5), with good prospects of benefit from it.

CHAPTER NINE

Tinnitus: Vertigo: Ménière's Disorder

TINNITUS

This most distressing symptom is characterised by the patient's experiencing noises in the ears. These noises are not heard in response to any outside stimulus and they are heard only by the patient.

The noises, which may occur in one or both ears, may take the form of humming, whistling, ringing, rushing or screeching sounds; they may occur at any time, and may vary in intensity. The noises are almost always worse at night.

There may be accompanying deafness, e.g. presbycusis (deafness of ageing), and sometimes there may be an ear condition present such as otosclerosis or otitis media. More often no cause is found.

Treatment is disappointing. Tranquilliser drugs may make the patient less aware of the noise. Any other noise which is going on in the environment at the same time may help to occupy the hearing in the affected ear and make the noise seem less loud. In recent years, tinnitus maskers have become available. These little devices look just like small post-aural hearing aids but emit a constant noise which drowns out the patient's own tinnitus. Some patients find this very helpful, but many do not.

Patients afflicted with this symptom need sympathetic advice and reassurance.

VERTIGO

The term describes the false sensation (hallucination) of movement experienced by a patient. It is a most distressing symptom and may be accompanied by nausea and vomiting as well as by other symptoms of ear disease such as deafness or tinnitus. The feeling of movement is exactly the same as the feeling after being on a round-about.

Maintenance of balance is a complicated action: in health the brain receives information from a number of sources, the eyes, the lateral semicircular canals and the muscles and joints (proprioceptive information). A disorder of any of these sources of input may result in the brain's receiving a false idea of position or posture and will give rise to a feeling of vertigo.

Causes

These include labyrinthitis, Ménière's disorder, following ear surgery, or after taking certain drugs such as streptomycin.

Conditions which affect the vestibular nerve or the vestibular pathways, such as acoustic neuroma and multiple sclerosis, may lead to complaints of vertigo by the patient.

Osteoarthritis of the cervical spine is another fairly common cause of vertigo.

Acoustic neuroma: The internal auditory canal is the name given to a short tube about 1cm in length on the medial side of the temporal bone (p. 29). Three important nerves pass through this canal, namely the acoustic, the vestibular and the facial. The internal auditory canal may be the site at which a tumour called an acoustic neuroma may develop. Contrary to what might be expected the tumour usually grows on the *vestibular* nerve. It is a benign tumour but as it enlarges it presses on the auditory nerve giving rise to gradually increasing deafness and frequently tinnitus. By virtue of its position, as it enlarges it will eventually press on vital centres in the brainstem and may be fatal. Before this terminal stage is reached other cranial nerves will be affected: there may be weakness of the facial muscles or, if the trigeminal nerve is affected, the face may be numb.

The unilateral deafness is perceptive in nature and specialised hearing tests can confirm that it is the nerve of hearing which is affected. *Caloric tests* will demonstrate impaired function of the lateral semicircular canal on the same side as the deafness.

Radiographic examination of the internal auditory canals may show widening and perhaps some erosion of bone on the affected side due to the enlarging tumour expanding the bony canal. A CT scan can demonstrate accurately the tumour, giving information regarding its size and position.

Treatment is surgical and such operations are usually carried out in special centres by a neurosurgeon and an ENT surgeon working together.

CALORIC TESTS

Caloric tests provide information about the parts of the inner ear responsible for balance (labyrinth). These tests work by virtue of the fact that the lateral semicircular canal lies close to the surface in the mastoid antrum. By changing the temperature in the ear canal using warm or cold water or air, the temperature of the air inside the middle ear and mastoid is altered. This in turn alters the temperature of the fluid in the lateral semicircular canal (endolymph) and sets up convection currents. As the endolymph moves, the sensory nerve endings are stimulated and this induces regular rhythmic eye movements (nystagmus). The eyes move slowly to one side (slow phase) with a fast flick back to the midline (fast phase). The duration of the nystagmus following a standard stimulation is related to the function of the labyrinth.

Method: The patient lies comfortably supine with the head supported and flexed at 30° to the horizontal. Flexing the head has the effect of making the lateral semicircular canal vertical. Therefore the caloric effects brought about by changing the temperature of the endolymph will have their greatest impact.

The ears are checked to make sure the meatus is not blocked by wax and that there is no tympanic membrane perforation. The patient's clothing is protected by waterproof drapes or towels and a receiver, for example a kidney dish, is placed beneath the ear to collect the water as it runs out.

The original caloric tests involved irrigating each ear separately with warm water at 30° C (cold irrigation) and 44° C (warm irrigation) for exactly 40 seconds.

The patient is asked to keep his eyes open and to look at the fixed spot on the ceiling directly in his line of vision. The exact duration of the nystagmus is then measured with a stop-watch. The results are recorded and the function of the patient's labyrinth on one side compared with the function on the other side. In this way impaired labyrinthine function on one side may be demonstrated as in Ménière's disorder or an acoustic neuroma.

In practice the exact duration of the nystagmus is difficult to measure because it is hard to be certain when the nystagmus is actually finished. The nystagmus may be measured electronically using an electronystagmograph (ENG). This machine relies on the fact that when the eyes look straight ahead there is a tiny difference in the electrical charge between the front and the back of the eyeball and this can be easily detected using electrodes placed on the skin near the eye. As the patient looks from one side to the other and the eye moves, the electrical charge alters slightly and these changes can be recorded. A caloric induced nystagmus gives a recording which is represented in Figure 9/1 which shows the slow phase of the nystagmus and the fast flick back to the midline (fast phase). Instead of recording the duration of the nystagmus the slope of the slow phase of the nystagmus is measured and this gives an accurate indication of the function of the labyrinth.

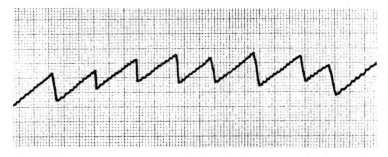

Fig. 9/1 Electronystagmography (ENG): Caloric testing, irrigating the left ear with warm water (44 C). The fast phase of the nystagmus is to the left (downward in this tracing)

MÉNIÈRE'S DISORDER

This comprises three main symptoms namely deafness, vertigo and tinnitus. The disease tends to occur in adult life and affects females more than males.

The underlying abnormality is known to be a rise in pressure of the endolymph causing dilatation of the endolymph-filled membranous labyrinth (see Fig. 4/5) with consequent distortion of the delicate inner ear membranes. It is this distortion which gives rise to the symptoms.

The exact reason for this rise in pressure is uncertain but it may be due to the fact that the rate of endolymph production is too great or the rate of re-absorption in the endolymphatic duct or sac is too small, leading to a gradual increase in the volume of endolymph in the inner ear.

The disease is characterised by episodes of rotatory vertigo which may be so severe that they cause the patient to fall to the ground, to feel nauseated and to vomit. For many patients the attack is preceded by a feeling of fullness in the affected ear and by worsening of the tinnitus along with deterioration in the hearing. Usually the disease starts in one ear, but in many patients the second ear will ultimately be affected.

Acute attacks usually last a few hours but it may be some days before the patient feels well enough to resume normal activity. As the attack subsides, so may the hearing and tinnitus improve. The hearing loss may thus appear to fluctuate but the tendency is for the hearing to gradually diminish with successive attacks. Initially, the hearing loss is predominantly in the low tones but later it comes to affect the middle and high tones. Distortion of hearing may be a prominent feature.

Such attacks usually occur in clusters, interspersed by varying periods of good health which may lead the patient and his doctor to believe that the condition has been cured. This fact makes the evaluation of the effectiveness of any treatment very difficult.

Treatment of the acute attack
If the patient has severe vertigo and feels sick he will certainly prefer to lie down quite still with the affected ear downward. Vomiting may be controlled by administration of an anti-emetic by mouth, by suppository or by injection.

Surgical treatment
In some cases the insertion of a grommet helps. Many patients say that their attacks of vertigo are immediately preceded by a feeling of fullness or of rising pressure within the ear. Such patients are often helped dramatically by the insertion of a grommet which equalises middle ear pressure to that of the atmosphere.

ULTRASOUND
The lateral semicircular canal is exposed surgically by a cortical mastoidectomy approach and the bone overlying the canal is thinned using a drill. The ultrasound probe is then applied over the semi-circular canal for a number of minutes. The sensitivity of the vestib-ular apparatus is gradually lessened and eventually abolished, with

preservation of hearing. For some patients this is a very effective method of controlling the symptoms of Ménière's disorder.

SACCUS DECOMPRESSION

This has already been referred to in the anatomy section (p. 34). Essentially it consists of exposing the endolymphatic sac by a cortical mastoidectomy approach and drilling away some bone in the region of the posterior fossa dura, and incising the sac to allow excess endolymph to drain away. A tiny tube is often inserted into the sac to keep the opening patent and to allow the endolymph to continue draining.

It should be possible to preserve the hearing by this method. There is an increasing tendency to attempt to do these various endolymph drainage procedures early in the course of the disease and so avoid the progressive sensori-neural hearing loss seen in the later stages of the disease.

LABYRINTHECTOMY

When the patient is incapacitated by vertigo with little or no useful residual hearing, the remaining function of the inner ear may be eliminated by labyrinthectomy.

The membranous labyrinth may be destroyed by removing the footplate of the stapes, draining away the perilymph and then pulling out the labyrinth with a pair of fine forceps. Alternatively the labyrinth may be removed using the electric cutting drill.

NERVE SECTION

More rarely the eighth cranial nerve or the vestibular division of this nerve may be cut by a neurosurgical approach.

Long-term medical treatment

A multitude of treatment regimes have been proposed and tried. These include a salt-free diet, preparations designed to reduce the amount of endolymph produced and preparations which improve the blood supply to the inner ear to increase the rate at which the endolymph is re-absorbed. Alternatively the long-term use of labyrinthine sedatives such as prochlorperazine (Stemetil) may be employed. Some patients may be taught special head and neck exercises by the physiotherapist, and for a number of patients these are helpful.

Section Two – The Nose and Sinuses

CHAPTER TEN

Anatomy and Physiology

Most people think of the nose as the part which appears on the face
– the external nose. Behind this external nose lies the nasal cavity
which is divided by the midline nasal septum into two portions.

The *paranasal sinuses* are air–containing cavities which lie adjacent
to, and communicate with, each nasal cavity.

EXTERNAL NOSE (Fig. 10/1a)

This structure is covered by skin and has a skeleton composed partly
of flexible cartilage. Each *nasal bone* is joined to the frontal process
of the maxilla and forms the upper part of the nasal skeleton. The
remainder of the skeleton of the nose is composed of *lateral cartilages*
and *alar cartilages* which form the lateral margin of the nostril or
anterior nares.

The profile of the nose is maintained by the edge of the nasal
septum to which the other cartilages are attached. This edge of the
septum is easily felt in one's own nose.

The free anterior edge of the nasal septum which lies between the
left and right nostrils is reinforced by parts of the alar cartilages and
is known as the *columella*.

The opening into each nasal cavity is known as the *vestibule*, which
is lined by ordinary skin bearing hairs known as *vibrissae*. These act
as a filter to trap dust particles.

Septum (Fig. 10/1b)

The nasal septum forms the party wall between the left and right
nostrils. It is composed of a skeleton of thin bone posteriorly (ethmoid bone superiorly and the vomer inferiorly) and a sheet of flexible
cartilage anteriorly. The cartilage and bone are covered by a thin
layer of tough fibrous tissue known as perichondrium and periosteum

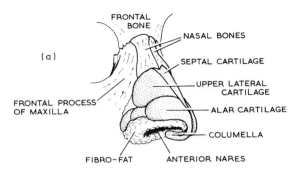

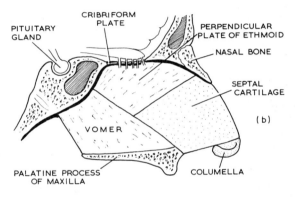

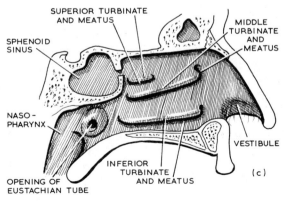

Fig. 10/1 The nose. (a) The external nose; (b) The nasal septum; (c) The turbinates; also showing the relationship of the nasal cavity to the ear via the Eustachian tube, and the nasopharynx

respectively. This fibrous covering layer is closely bound to the cartilage and bone and contains blood vessels which nourish these structures. The septum is covered by a mucous membrane containing mucous glands and bearing cilia. The nasal septum is richly supplied with nerves and blood vessels.

The nasal septum theoretically lies in the midline but commonly deviates slightly to one side or the other. Sometimes this deflection is so severe that one nostril becomes blocked. The septum may then need to be straightened surgically (see submucous resection). The nasal septum helps to maintain the profile of the nose, and removal of too much cartilage from the septum may result in collapse of the nose.

Each nasal cavity is larger than one thinks: the floor of the nose corresponds to the roof of the mouth and therefore each nasal cavity is about 8cm in length. The height from the floor to the roof is about 5cm. The roof of the nose is formed by the *cribriform plate* (Fig. 10/1b). This is a thin plate of bone perforated by the terminal branches of the olfactory nerve, serving the sense of smell, and separates the nasal cavity from the anterior cranial fossa containing the frontal lobes of the brain.

The medial wall of each nasal cavity is formed by the nasal septum which is usually fairly flat and smooth. The lateral wall is not flat (Fig. 10/1c). Into each nasal cavity project three ridges – the turbinates: the *inferior turbinate* which lies nearest to the floor of the nose and is the largest; the *middle turbinate*, and the *superior turbinate* which is the smallest of the three and is situated nearest the roof of the nose. Beneath each turbinate is a recess known as a *meatus* each of which is named after the turbinate above it.

These meati, or recesses, are important because the paranasal sinuses and the nasolacrimal duct open into them. Each sinus or group of sinuses communicates with the nasal cavity through a separate opening or ostium, like a series of rooms opening into a corridor. Most of the sinuses open into the middle meatus beneath the middle turbinate.

The posterior outlet of each nasal cavity is known as the *posterior choana* and is about the same size as the thumb print of the patient concerned. Behind the posterior choanae is the nasopharynx which is the uppermost part of the pharynx and extends down to the level of the soft palate. Into each lateral wall of the nasopharynx protrudes the lower end of the Eustachian tube.

In children a collection of lymphoid tissue known as the *adenoid* lies on the posterior wall. The adenoid forms part of a protective ring of lymphoid tissue which encircles the upper air and food passages. The adenoid pad gradually enlarges through the early years of childhood to reach a maximum size at 6 or 7 years of age. It also enlarges in response to bouts of upper respiratory tract infection. Thereafter the adenoids become relatively smaller so that by the age of 11 or 12 years they may be barely visible.

SINUSES (Fig. 10/2)

The paranasal sinuses are air-containing cavities which lie adjacent to, and communicate with, the nasal cavity in a similar way that a series of rooms may lead on to a corridor. Just as each room has a door, so each sinus has an ostium. Each sinus is lined by the same type of ciliated columnar epithelium which lines the nose. Each sinus has its own opening or ostium except in the case of the ethmoid

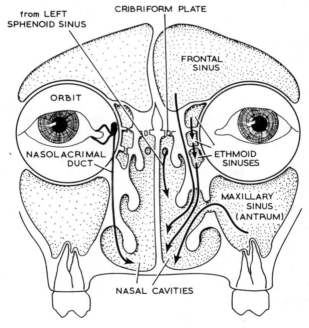

Fig. 10/2 The paranasal sinuses

sinuses where a small number of ethmoid air cells may communicate with each other and then share a common opening into the cavity.

Maxillary sinus

This is commonly known as the *antrum* and lies lateral to the nasal cavity behind the cheek, one in either side. Inferiorly it is related to the roots of the teeth of the upper jaw so the sinus may become involved in dental infection. The ceiling of the antrum corresponds to the floor of the orbit and consists of only a very thin sheet of bone. Disease which involves the antrum may therefore spread upward and involve the eye and any surgeon who operates on the maxillary sinus must bear this important relationship in mind.

The maxillary sinus ostium lies halfway up the side wall of the sinus, beneath the middle turbinate, so any secretions which are produced in the sinus have to be wafted upward towards the ostium by the action of the cilia which cover the surface of the lining epithelium. Any disease process which blocks the ostium or interferes with the action of the cilia will result in stagnation of secretions in the sinus with subsequent infection.

Ethmoid sinuses

The ethmoid sinuses are a collection of 10 or more smaller air cells lying between the nasal cavity and the medial border (or corner) of the eye, above the level of the maxillary antrum. The ethmoid cells are usually divided into groups called anterior, middle and posterior, and the majority open into the middle meatus of the nose.

Ethmoid infections are particularly likely to occur in children, and orbital complications may develop due to the proximity of the eye.

The lining membrane of the ethmoid sinuses is only loosely attached to the underlying bony walls so nasal polyps, which are oedematous swellings of the lining membrane, are especially likely to develop in the ethmoids before prolapsing down into the nose.

The close relationship of the ethmoids to the orbit means· that great care must be taken during operations to avoid damage to the contents of the orbit with resultant blindness.

Frontal sinus

These sinuses, one on each side, lie above and medial to the eye, in the frontal bone. There is tremendous variation in the shape and size of the frontal sinus, and for any individual the configuration of the outline of the frontal sinuses, as seen on a radiograph, is as characteristic as a finger-print.

The frontal sinus drains into the anterior end of the middle meatus of the nose via a duct which is sometimes narrow and which may become blocked and result in infection or, alternatively, in accumulation of secretions and consequent expansion of the sinus (mucocele).

Sphenoid sinus

The sphenoid sinus lies beyond the uppermost part of the nose posteriorly. It is usually divided into two by a bony septum. Like other sinuses the sphenoid sinus may become infected or the lining membrane may become thickened and polypoidal.

The sphenoid sinus lies in front of the pituitary gland and forms a convenient route for operations to remove the pituitary gland (transsphenoidal hypophysectomy).

BLOOD SUPPLY OF THE NOSE (Fig. 10/3)

The nasal cavities and the paranasal sinuses are supplied with branches of the external and internal carotid arteries.

The maxillary artery is a branch of the external carotid artery and its branches supply most of the nasal septum and the lower part of

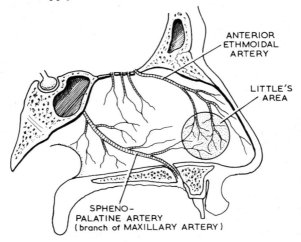

Fig. 10/3 The blood supply to the nose

the lateral wall of the nose. The superior labial artery, a branch of the facial artery, supplies the anterior half of the nasal septum and anastomoses with one of the branches of the maxillary artery to form a small plexus of blood vessels from which bleeding readily occurs. The area where these small blood vessels come together is called *Little's Area*. The other part of the nasal septum, the roof of the nose and the upper half of the side wall of the nose are supplied by the anterior and posterior ethmoidal arteries – branches of the internal carotid artery. Bleeding from these vessels is seen above the level of the middle turbinate.

The veins of the nose form a cavernous plexus beneath the mucous membrane and from here blood drains into the facial veins, the ophthalmic veins and directly to veins on the surface of the frontal lobe of the brain. The importance of this lies in the fact that a severe sinus infection may sometimes result in orbital or intracranial complications as the result of the spread of sepsis via the veins.

The blood supply to the nasal mucous membrane is controlled by the *autonomic nervous system*. Sympathetic nerve fibres maintain a constant tone in the vessels and interruption of the nerve supply, e.g. by cervical sympathectomy, will sometimes cause a stuffy nose. Parasympathetic fibres cause vasodilatation and division of the parasympathetic supply will cause vasoconstriction and diminution of nasal secretions.

PHYSIOLOGY

Breathing
When a person breathes in through the nose the column of air is broken up by the turbinates and passes into each of the meati thus helping to clear away the mucus which is expelled from the sinus.

The turbinates therefore increase the surface area of the nasal mucosa, improving the efficiency with which incoming air is warmed and moistened.

The nasal mucous membrane is composed of ciliated columnar epithelium. Mucus is constantly being produced and moistens the incoming air which is then warmed as it comes into contact with the highly vascular lining of the nose. Particulate matter in the atmosphere sticks to this moist surface and the cilia then transport this mucous blanket to the back of the nose and into the nasopharynx. This mucus then passes unnoticed down the back of the throat and is swallowed.

Olfaction (smelling)

Branches of the olfactory nerve enter the nasal cavity from the brain through the roof of the nose. The nerve fibres pass through tiny holes in the cribriform plate (see p. 87) from whence they are distributed to an area of the nasal mucosa high in the nose. Any disease process which prevents air from reaching the olfactory area high in the nose, such as oedema which accompanies the common cold, or nasal polypi, will result in loss of sense of smell, anosmia.

Some viruses, for example those which cause influenza, may attack the olfactory nerve endings and result in permanent loss of sense of smell, as will head injuries which may cause a shearing of the nerve fibres.

CHAPTER ELEVEN

Epistaxis

Epistaxis is the technical term to describe bleeding from the nasal cavity and it is a very common ENT symptom. In children and young adults the bleeding point is usually in the nasal septum from an area where a number of blood vessels meet and anastomose known as Little's Area (see p. 91). The bleeding is often caused by minor trauma such as picking the nose and is usually easily controlled by firm pressure, i.e. by squeezing the nose.

TREATMENT

The patient should be reassured that all will be well: always remember that a little blood can look a lot, so the patient is bound to be anxious if he thinks he has lost a lot of blood. He should be seated upright in a firm-backed chair with the head bent slightly forward. The soft part of the nose is then pinched firmly between thumb and forefinger. The patient should breathe through his mouth and be told not to swallow any blood which may trickle down the back of the throat. Instead he should spit the blood out into a bowl or paper tissues. In most cases the bleeding will have stopped after 10 minutes.

If nose bleeds are persistently troublesome the offending blood vessel may be identified and cauterised under local anaesthetic using a caustic chemical such as silver nitrate or trichloracetic acid, or with the electrocautery.

Sometimes simple pressure applied from the outside is not effective. This is particularly likely in middle aged and elderly patients who may have hypertension (high blood pressure). In these patients the bleeding often comes from farther back in the nose where the blood vessels may be brittle, due to atherosclerosis. The natural process of coagulation and cessation of bleeding occurs less readily because the vessel wall is unable to contract.

The flow of blood will stop if pressure can be applied over the bleeding point and the conventional method is to pack the nasal cavity with 1.25cm ($\frac{1}{2}$in) BIPP Gauze.

Method of packing

The patient's clothing is protected with a mackintosh or towels. After gently dilating the nares with a nasal speculum, the surgeon removes any blood clot from the nose with a nasal sucker and looks for the source of bleeding with a good light. It may be impossible to see the bleeding point if it is a long way back. The nasal cavity is gently but firmly packed with a length of 1.25cm ($\frac{1}{2}$in) BIPP Gauze. This has the advantage of being antiseptic and, as it will not adhere to the nasal mucous membrane, it may be easily removed after 24 hours. The loose ends of the pack are secured at the front of the nose by being knotted together. If this is not done, loose ends may tend to fall down the back of the nose. This will make the patient retch, the pack will become dislodged and the bleeding will restart.

Subsequently the patient is admitted, placed in bed and sedated to relieve the anxiety. Many patients seem to have a high blood pressure when first seen but this is often due merely to anxiety and will quickly settle with bed rest and sedation once the bleeding has stopped.

As an alternative a special inflatable rubber balloon may be inserted into the nose and inflated to exert pressure on the bleeding point.

If the nose is completely occluded by packing, the patient will be unable to breathe through his nose and will have to breathe solely through his mouth. The mouth will become dry and uncomfortable unless careful attention is paid to regular mouth care and teeth brushing. Extra fluids must be given by mouth to make up for fluid lost in this way.

The packing or the balloon is removed after 24 hours. If bleeding recurs the packing may have to be reinserted.

If the patient loses a lot of blood then blood should be taken for grouping and cross-matching; an intravenous infusion of normal saline should be set up and the patient given a blood transfusion as soon as the blood is available.

Once the epistaxis has been controlled it may be necessary to consider other conditions, such as coagulation defects, which may need to be fully investigated and treated if the bleeding does not stop in response to simple measures. If the patient's blood pressure is consistently elevated then the advice of a physician should be sought.

Surgical management

If the bleeding is severe or prolonged and does not respond to the measures already described then it may be necessary to ligate the artery responsible. The maxillary artery and its branches lie behind the maxillary antrum so may be approached via a Caldwell-Luc type of incision (see p. 104) and the vessels occluded by metal clips. Alternatively the external carotid artery may be ligated in the neck above the level at which the common carotid artery divides into external and internal carotid arteries.

On the rare occasions when the bleeding comes from high up in the nose, the anterior ethmoidal artery may be ligated as it runs alongside the medial wall of the orbit (Fig. 11/1).

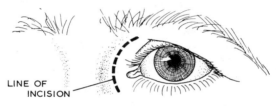

LINE OF
INCISION

Fig. 11/1 Incision for ligating the anterior ethmoidal artery

NURSING MANAGEMENT

A patient with severe epistaxis is an emergency admission. He is likely to be very anxious and will need reassurance from both the medical and nursing staff.

If the bleeding cannot be controlled by electrocautery to the offending vessel in the nose, a pack or epistaxis balloon is put into either one or both nostrils.

REQUIREMENTS FOR PACKING THE NOSE
  BIPP pack
  Vomit bowl for patient to spit blood into
  Tilley's forceps (see Fig. 1/1)
  Plastic aprons for both doctor and patient
  Local anaesthetic spray, e.g. 5% cocaine
  Gauze bolster and tape

REQUIREMENTS IF A BALLOON IS USED
Epistaxis balloon or Foley's catheter
BIPP Gauze
Syringe to inflate balloon with air
KY jelly
Protection for doctor and patient
Vomit bowl
Local anaesthetic spray
Gauze bolster and tape

Nursing care

1. The airway should be cleared through the mouth. The nurse must make sure the pack has not fallen down into the naso-pharynx or, in the case of a balloon, that it is not causing an obstruction.
2. If the bleeding has been severe, replacement of fluid by intra-venous infusion or even transfusion, may be necessary. The nurse will have to monitor the fluid intake and output.
3. The patient will be on bed rest and all general nursing care will be necessary, including pressure area care.
4. Sedation will almost certainly be required and this will be pre-scribed by the doctor. In addition, the nurse will need to spend time with the patient giving strong reassurance.
5. Four-hourly observations (temperature, pulse and respiration) and blood pressure will need to be recorded until the patient's condition becomes stable.
6. Mouth care. This is important because the patient has to breathe through the mouth and so it becomes very dry. The patient should be given regular mouthwashes and he may wish to brush his teeth gently.
7. Deep vein thrombosis is always a possibility when a patient is on bed rest. The nurse should encourage the patient to carry out simple foot exercises; if he is unable to do them himself, the nurse should carry out regular passive movements. Thrombo–embolic stockings may be worn to prevent thrombosis occurring.

Nursing problems

(a) Further bleeding may occur and the nurse needs to be on the alert for possible indications such as fresh bleeding from the nose, and spitting or vomiting of swallowed blood. A rising pulse rate or pallor should also raise suspicion that there is bleeding.

(b) An infection in the nose, due to the balloon or the packing, may become apparent. As with possible bleeding, the nurse must be alert to any signs of an impending infection, such as unpleasant odour, pyrexia or pain, and inform the doctor, who may prescribe an antibiotic.

(c) In spite of careful nursing a deep vein thrombosis may occur. The nurse must be aware of this and watch for the warning signs – inflamed veins in the calf, pain on dorsiflexion, pyrexia. She should inform the doctor. The foot of the bed should be raised and the patient further reassured.

(d) If a blood transfusion is necessary, the nurse must observe the patient for any signs of a reaction. These include fever, perhaps with rigors, and nausea and vomiting. These reactions are not uncommon and may be due to the presence of white blood cell antibodies formed as a result of previous transfusions or pregnancies.

More severe reactions due to haemolysis of the transfused red cells give rise to symptoms which include pain and heat along the vein receiving the transfusion, facial flushing, fever and rigors, severe loin pain and a feeling of constriction in the chest. These may be followed by hypotension, shock and even by death. At the first sign of any of these, the transfusion should be stopped and the doctor informed at once.

Mobilisation and discharge

(a) If there is no further bleeding the pack may be removed after 24–48 hours. For method of removal see page 105.

(b) The patient may sit in a chair later on the day of the removal of the pack and start to become mobile round the ward and self-caring the next day.

(c) When he is discharged he should be advised to take things easy, not to blow his nose or pick any crust off. Antibiotics or Naseptin cream may need to be continued for several days.

Follow-up may be needed if hypertension has been diagnosed as the cause of epistaxis – such appointments should be made with the appropriate outpatient clinic before discharge from the ward. Similarly, if a blood coagulation disorder has been found to be the cause.

CHAPTER TWELVE

Sinusitis

Acute sinusitis is inflammation of the lining mucosa of any of the paranasal sinuses. It almost always follows an acute inflammation of the nose (rhinitis) of which the most common cause is a cold. This is because the mucosa lining the nose and sinuses is in continuity. Acute sinusitis may also follow trauma or dental sepsis. Sometimes jumping into a river or a swimming pool without pinching the nose may force water into the sinuses giving rise to inflammation.

The acute inflammatory process in the mucosa causes the surface of the mucous membrane to become coated with fibrin and exudate containing pus cells. The mucous glands will produce an increased amount of mucus which then mixes with the pus cells to form muco-pus. The sticky fibrin seals off the natural ostium ('the door closes') and the pus becomes trapped in the sinus.

As the pressure of the pus in the sinus rises, bone necrosis may occur and, rarely, septicaemia may develop. Infection and thrombosis in the venous channels may spread to the meninges (the covering layers of the brain) and meningitis may occur with brain abscesses. While this may be fatal, thankfully it is now rare because antibiotics are used readily to treat sinusitis.

CLINICAL FEATURES

The patient has usually had a cold for a few days but just as it should have been improving, the condition worsens. The nose becomes more blocked and the nasal discharge becomes thicker. The patient feels generally unwell, feverish and may have pain in his cheeks which is made worse on bending forward. There may be a headache on waking but this will clear as the nasal congestion, which has become worse through lying, clears when the patient is up and about.

The patient may look unwell and breathes through his mouth because his nose is blocked. The temperature is raised. Examination usually shows the skin of the nasal vestibule to be red while the nasal mucous membrane itself is red and congested. There may be visible pus in the nose. Pressure on the cheek is usually painful although the cheek itself may not be swollen.

The diagnosis may be confirmed by finding a raised white cell count and the radiographic appearance of the sinuses. Nasal swabs are seldom helpful because the swab usually becomes contaminated with other bacteria within the nasal passages and therefore gives no useful information regarding the pathogenic bacteria causing the sinus infection.

TREATMENT

1. The patient should rest in bed, preferably propped up with pillows to relieve some of the nasal congestion which would result from lying flat. Fluids should be encouraged, also a light diet.
2. Regular mouthwashes and teeth cleaning will help to keep the oral cavity healthy.
3. Paper tissues should be used to blow the nose. These are collected in a suitable bag and subsequently burnt.
4. Simple analgesia, such as aspirin or paracetamol, may be helpful in relieving discomfort.
5. Nasal decongestants, e.g. 1% ephedrine nose drops, should be given to shrink down the lining membrane of the nose allowing the natural ostium of the sinus to open. This will allow the infected material in the sinus to drain away.
6. An antibiotic, such as amoxycillin, starting with an intramuscular injection and continuing orally, should be prescribed.

Antral washout (Fig. 12/1)
If, in spite of the above conservative treatment, the symptoms and clinical signs persist then further measures must be taken in the form of sinus washout. This procedure:

1. Confirms the presence of infection in the antrum.
2. Allows a pure specimen of pus to be sent to the laboratory for bacteriological examination, which will enable the correct antibiotic to be prescribed.
3. Speeds recovery through irrigating the sinus and washing out the infected material.

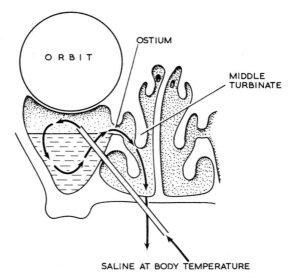

Fig. 12/1 To illustrate an antral washout, showing the position
of the cannula

Careful explanation, reassurance and an air of confidence on the
part of the doctor and the nurse will permit the procedure to be
carried out under local anaesthetic in the majority of adult patients.
In children, or if the patient is unduly apprehensive, the operation
may require to be carried out under general anaesthesia.

LOCAL ANAESTHESIA
The patient should be seated in a chair where he may be observed
carefully in case there are any reactions to the local anaesthetic (see
p. 19).

The front of the nasal passages are first sprayed with a solution of
local anaesthetic such as 10% cocaine or a mixture of lignocaine and
adrenaline. This has the effect not only of anaesthetising the lining
of the nose but will also shrink the nasal lining thereby allowing the
surgeon a better view of the opening of the inferior meatus.

The maxillary sinus can be punctured easily through the lateral
wall of the nasal cavity in the inferior meatus below the inferior
turbinate for at this point the bone is very thin. Therefore only the
inferior meatus needs to be anaesthetised and this can be done using

a fine flexible metal probe the end of which is covered with cotton wool. Local anaesthetic in the form of 10% cocaine hydrochloride solution or 25% cocaine paste is applied to the cotton wool and the probe is gently inserted beneath the anterior end of the inferior turbinate and into the inferior meatus where it remains for 10–15 minutes.

REQUIREMENTS FOR THE ANTRAL WASHOUT
1. Waterproof sheeting and/or towels to keep the patient's clothing clean and dry.
2. A sterile trochar and cannula, Higginson syringe and tubing with a suitable connector which will fit the cannula.
3. Irrigating solution, e.g. sterile normal saline at body temperature, 37°C.
4. A Thudicum nasal speculum (see Fig. 1/1, p. 2).
5. A bowl into which the washings can be collected.
6. Specimen bottles and the relevant pathology forms.
7. Plenty of paper towels or tissues.
8. A mouthwash for the patient to use at the conclusion of the procedure.

There should also be a suitable source of light for the surgeon – a headlight or a head mirror and bull's-eye lamp.

METHOD
Some surgeons perform a sinus washout with the patient sitting while others prefer the patient to be lying.

The patient's clothing should be covered by the waterproof drapes; the probes which carry the local anaesthetic are removed from the nose.

The surgeon checks that the trochar and cannula fit together and come apart easily. The tip of the trochar and cannula are inserted beneath the inferior turbinate until the surgeon feels that he is in the correct place. The handle of the trochar is then angled so that the tip of the trochar is pointing directly towards the maxillary sinus. By exerting firm but gentle pressure the side wall of the nose is punctured and the tip of the trochar and cannula enter the sinus. Puncturing the side wall of the nose is usually accompanied by a rather alarming crunching noise as the thin bone is broken – a few well-chosen words of reassurance will usually put the patient at ease. The trochar is removed from the cannula which is then gently advanced further into the antrum. The Higginson syringe is filled with the irrigating solution by the nurse and the tubing connected to the cannula. The patient is asked to hold the bowl (if he is not able to do this, then a nurse will) and instructed to bend his head forward and to breathe in and out gently through the open mouth. The bulb of the Higginson's syringe is gently squeezed, the solution passing through the cannula into the antrum and out through the natural ostium (Fig. 12/1). The fluid then drips from the nose into the bowl that is held either by the patient or the nurse. Any pus or infected material irrigated from the sinus may be retrieved from the bowl, placed in a specimen bottle and sent, fully labelled, to the laboratory.

When the returned irrigating fluid is clear, the tubing is disconnected and the cannula gently withdrawn. If both sinuses are to be washed out, the procedure is repeated on the second side.

Once the procedure has been completed, the patient should be given a mouthwash, and advised to sit quietly until he is fully recovered and able to go home. A relative or friend should accompany him.

An attack of sinusitis will normally resolve if adequately treated. The natural ostium re-opens and the ciliated lining of the sinus returns to its normal healthy state. The cilia waft the mucus towards the ostium which in the case of the maxillary antrum is halfway up the medial wall of the antrum. Gravity, therefore, has little or no part to play in the drainage of secretions from the sinus into the nose and this drainage is achieved almost entirely by the action of the ciliated lining.

If the infection in the antrum fails to resolve in response to the treatment already described, it may either be because the ostium has failed to open properly or the action of the cilia has not returned to normal. Under these circumstances it will be helpful to create a new drainage opening for the sinus.

Intranasal antrostomy
This is a surgically created opening in the inferior meatus of the nose, the opening lying almost level with the floor of the sinus so that secretions may easily drain into the nose with the help of gravity.

METHOD
Under general anaesthesia the opening is made, using punch forceps, by removing an area of thin bone approximately 2 × 1cm level with

the floor of the nose. Before making the opening the mucosa of the inferior meatus should be painted with a vasoconstrictor such as cocaine paste to reduce the amount of bleeding which occurs. If bleeding is troublesome, the nose may be packed at the end of the operation with 2.5cm (1in) ribbon gauze, impregnated with petroleum jelly or BIPP.

These packs are removed the following morning, usually by the nurse. Once the packs are removed ephedrine nose drops and inhalations with menthol and eucalyptus will help clear away any dried secretions, blood or crusts in the nose. These should be continued at home for 10 days.

After making an intranasal antrostomy it will be easily possible to irrigate the sinus afterwards using a Higginson syringe and a curved metal cannula. Many patients with long-standing sinus infection may be taught to carry out this procedure themselves.

CHRONIC SINUSITIS

If acute sinusitis does not completely clear and the mucous membrane does not return to its original healthy state, chronic sinusitis results. Just as the body's defences are gaining the upper hand the position can be reversed and a new infection gains the upper hand. With successive waves of infection the mucous membrane becomes thickened and scarred with areas of fibrosis; the normal healthy thin lining of ciliated columnar epithelium becomes totally replaced by a tough polypoid lining. Cilia are greatly reduced in number allowing sinus secretions to collect in the sinus and become stagnant, creating more infection.

It becomes increasingly difficult for the sinus to drain as the ostium becomes scarred, and antibiotics become less effective because they are unable to penetrate the thick lining membrane to reach the infected sinus contents. Chronic sinusitis can lead to ill-health with long-standing nasal obstruction and discharge with discomfort or pains in the face and head giving rise to a general feeling of malaise.

All sinuses may be affected; often more than one sinus is affected at any one time although the maxillary antra are the most commonly involved.

Surgical treatment (Caldwell–Luc operation) (Fig. 12/2)
Chronic sinusitis may be relieved by complete stripping out of the diseased sinus lining. The best way to approach the maxillary antrum

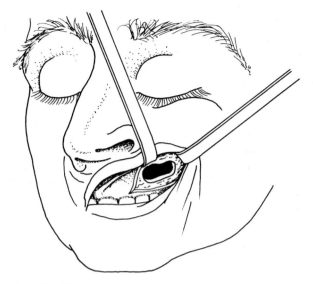

Fig. 12/2 Caldwell-Luc operation

surgically is through an incision above the upper teeth (or gum) and pushing the soft tissues of the cheek upwards to reveal the bony anterior wall of the sinus. (This method takes the name of a Caldwell-Luc operation because it was described by two men at roughly the same time – one was an American named Caldwell and the other a Frenchman called Luc.) An opening is then made in the bony anterior wall of the sinus and, under direct vision, the diseased lining of the sinus is stripped out. It may then be sent for histological examination.

To complete the operation and to improve subsequent drainage an intranasal antrostomy is made into the inferior meatus.

The incision may be loosely sutured or may be left to heal on its own. The nose may be packed as described for an intranasal antrostomy but on occasions the bleeding from the sinus itself may be so severe that the sinus has to be packed and the packing removed after 24 hours.

This approach to the maxillary antrum is useful in other respects, namely:

1. To evaluate and biopsy tumours of the antrum.

2. To approach the ethmoid sinuses in cases of nasal polyposis – transantral ethmoidectomy.
3. To approach and ligate the maxillary artery in cases of severe epistaxis.

POSTOPERATIVE ADVICE
It is not at all unusual for there to be a lot of oedema of the cheek postoperatively as a result of the manipulation and retraction during the operation. This will clear in a few days. Patients should be told not to poke the wound beneath the upper lip with their tongue or this could disrupt the wound and lead to a fistula forming. For the same reasons, upper dentures should not be worn until the wound has healed.

NURSING NOTES
The principles of nursing care following nasal surgery are discussed in Chapter 13.

CHAPTER THIRTEEN

Nursing Management for Nasal Surgery

This section will only comment on those specific points which the nurse should bear in mind when caring for patients undergoing surgery on the nose. The general use of the nursing process has been previously discussed in Chapter 2. Tables 13/1 and 13/2 show examples of postoperative care plans. The care plan should take into account the following:

PRE-OPERATIVE

1. All patients having nose operations should be free from infection, e.g. colds.
2. An explanation should be given to both patient and relatives as to what the operation entails. The patient should also be told that he will have packs in his nose after the operation and will have to breathe through his mouth. Most people like to know how long they are likely to remain in hospital.
3. Radiographic examination of the sinuses may be required.

POSTOPERATIVE

1. *Position of patient:* On return to the ward from the recovery ward, the patient will usually be lying on his side to help keep the airway clear and to prevent inhalation of blood.
2. *Ensuring a clear airway:* Following most nasal operations the nose will be packed with, for example, ribbon gauze, and there will be a square of gauze folded and taped across the bottom of the nose. The patient therefore has no option but to breathe through the mouth: the mouth must be kept clear of blood and secretions and suction may need to be used.
   If the patient is agitated and appears to be choking or retching

Table 13/1 Immediate postoperative care plan for a nasal operation

Problem	Goal/objective	Care/action	Evaluation
1. Possible airway obstruction due to pack slipping	Maintain clear airway	Nurse in lateral position Check mouth regularly for pack in throat	Pack(s) in position Airway clear
2. Possible shock from haemorrhage	Stable observations and no bleeding	$\frac{1}{2}$-hourly pulse; hourly blood pressure Check nasal bolster and the mouth for excessive bleeding Bed rest	Observations stable No bleeding – discontinue
3. Dry mouth	Clean moist tongue	Two-hourly mouthwashes and oral toilet	Clean fresh mouth
4. Pain	Keep patient pain-free	Postoperative medication as directed, or as needed	Comfortable postoperative evening

Table 13/2 Postoperative care plan for the morning following a nasal operation

Problem	Goal/objective	Care/action	Evaluation
1. Blocked nose 2. Possible epistaxis after removal of packs	Free nasal passages Control bleeding	Remove nasal packs Sit patient up Apply pressure to nostrils and ice pack on bridge of nose	Clearer nasal passage Bleeding stopped
3. Swollen nasal passages	Ease breathing through nose Prevent crusting in nostril	Menthol and eucalyptus inhalations and ephedrine nasal drops three times a day, or as prescribed by the surgeon	No crusting Able to breathe through nose

the nurse should suspect that the pack may have slipped backward into the pharynx. It may be possible to confirm this by looking into the patient's throat with a torch: the doctor should be informed at once. If the patient appears to be choking the nurse should remove the packing immediately. If only a small amount of packing has slipped backward into the pharynx, it may be possible to cut the piece off with a pair of scissors, otherwise the packing may have to be removed.

3. *Observations:* The pulse and blood pressure should be checked regularly and the patient observed for signs of fresh bleeding from the nose. A small amount of bleeding into the bolster may be anticipated; the bolster should be changed as necessary but kept in order to gauge the blood loss.

   Excessive bleeding may appear as fresh blood on the nasal bolster or as bleeding backward into the throat and then either spat out or vomited.

4. *Sedation:* Nasal packs can be quite distressing for some patients and sedation may be required. Patients often complain of headache and as soon as they are able to drink, simple analgesics such as paracetamol will suffice.

5. *Oral hygiene:* Mouthwashes, such as Thymol Glycerine Co., should be given frequently because the mouth will become very dry if the nose is packed and the patient has to breathe through his mouth. Sucking ice cubes is very soothing.

6. *Diet and fluids:* Provided the patient is not nauseated fluids may be started four hours after the operation and a normal diet resumed the following morning.

Removal of nasal packs

Nasal packs can be of different types: ribbon gauze impregnated with petroleum jelly, or BIPP; glove finger packs; or petroleum jelly gauze 'trousers'. When the surgeon writes the operation notes he should state the type of pack inserted and when it is to be removed; for most operations it is usually possible to remove the packs before breakfast the following morning. (The patient will also enjoy breakfast more if the packs are out.)

EQUIPMENT

A tray
Tilley's nasal dressing forceps (see Fig. 1/1, p. 2)
A kidney dish or similar bowl

Inco pad or plastic sheeting to protect patient's pyjamas in case
the nose bleeds
Some gauze squares to make a bolster
Adhesive tape to secure the bolster

METHOD
Removal of nasal packs is uncomfortable, so the nurse needs to
reassure the patient; she should encourage him to take regular deep
breaths through his mouth while the packs are being removed, one
side being done at a time. The patient's eyes usually water as the
lining membrane of the nose is stimulated.

Usually there will be some bleeding which settles quickly with
gentle pressure or with a small ice pack on the nose. Any blood
which goes down the back of the nose may be spat out into the dish.

Once all the packs are removed a piece of gauze swab is folded
and placed under the nose. It is held in place by adhesive tape to
the cheeks. It is expected that there will be a slight oozing of bloodstained fluid for a day or two so the bolster will need to be regularly
changed.

The patient is told *not* to blow his nose because this can start it
bleeding again.

This method of removing packs is also used after an epistaxis
which has required packing.

Inhalations
Steam inhalations, to which have been added menthol and eucalyptus
or something similar, are usually given to the patient to prevent
crusting inside the nose and may be started four to six hours after
the packs have been removed.

EQUIPMENT
5ml 2% menthol and eucalyptus
Small jug or Nelson inhaler
Bowl in which to stand jug
A waterproof cape
Towel
Hot water

METHOD
The jug is half filled with hot water. The menthol eucalyptus is
poured in and then the jug is placed firmly in the bowl. The nurse

takes the bowl to the patient and places it on a firm, stable surface such as the bedside table. The patient sits in a chair, the waterproof cape is placed round the shoulders, he places the towel over his head and leans over the jug, breathing first up one nostril and then the other. This may continue for about 10 minutes by which time the steam will have cooled. The nurse should remain with the patient until she is certain that he can manage with safety. *Remember*, the water used is hot and could scald the patient if the jug/inhaler tips over. Children must *never* be left at any time.

Nose drops (Fig. 13/1)

To administer nose drops the patient lies flat on his back (supine) on his bed. One pillow is tucked under his neck so that the head is back over the edge, i.e. in slight hyperextension. Two drops of 1% ephedrine are inserted into each nostril. The patient should remain in this position for five minutes to allow the ephedrine to have its effect on the nose, namely to reduce some of the swelling of the nasal mucosa which inevitably occurs after surgery. The head is then turned to each side for 30 seconds to encourage the distribution of the drops inside the nose.

NURSING PROBLEMS

1. Haemorrhage
2. Haematoma – septal (following SMR). This is caused by an accumulation of blood between the two layers of the septal mucosa. When the doctor examines the nose postoperatively he will see the widened septum. The haematoma must be drained.
3. Pyrexia
4. Infection of nose or sinuses

DISCHARGE AND CONVALESCENCE

Provided the patient is feeling well, and the nasal discharge is minimal, he may go home; this is usually two or three days after the operation. He should be given a supply of inhalations and drugs and carefully instructed in their use. Where necessary such instruction should be written out to avoid any misunderstanding. Such after-treatment should continue twice a day for 10 days. The patient is

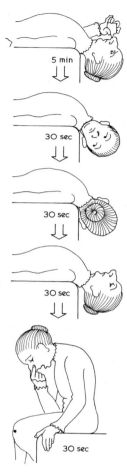

Fig. 13/1 Inserting nose drops

advised not to blow the nose hard for 10 days but rather to sniff
gently to clear the nose.

Most patients are able to return to work about 10 days after the
operation.

CHAPTER FOURTEEN

Submucous Resection: Nasal Polypectomy

SUBMUCOUS RESECTION (SMR) (Fig. 14/1)

The nasal septum is the party wall between the left and the right nasal cavities and in most normal noses lies in, or fairly near, the midline (see Fig. 10/1, p. 86).

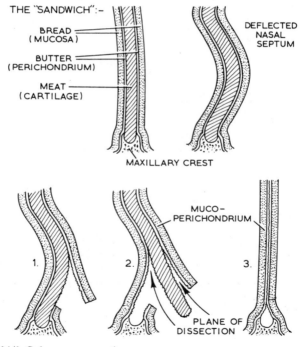

THE "SANDWICH":-

BREAD (MUCOSA)

BUTTER (PERICHONDRIUM)

MEAT (CARTILAGE)

DEFLECTED NASAL SEPTUM

MAXILLARY CREST

MUCO-PERICHONDRIUM

1.

2.

3.

PLANE OF DISSECTION

Fig. 14/1 Submucous resection

The septum may be either congenitally displaced and deviated to one side or deformed as a result of injury such as a punch on the nose. The deviation may be great enough to give rise to nasal obstruction, which is often worse on one side. If the patient is sufficiently bothered by his nasal blockage, then this may be corrected surgically by the operation of submucous resection of the nasal septum (SMR).

The operation is best understood by considering the nasal septum as a sandwich. The mucous membrane covering the septum is the 'bread' of the sandwich. The 'meat' of the sandwich corresponds with the cartilage which gives the septum support. Further posteriorly, the septal cartilage is replaced by thin bone. The cartilage is covered by a layer of perichondrium and this may be thought of as the butter in the sandwich (Fig. 14/1).

The aim of the operation is to remove the filling of the sandwich and to leave the two slices of bread and butter which will then stick to each other, in the midline.

An incision is made through the mucous membrane and perichondrium on one side of the septum, and through this incision the deviated cartilaginous and bony parts of the septum are filleted out.

If all the cartilage were to be removed then the shape of the nose would eventually collapse; to prevent this happening a strip of cartilage is left along the dorsum of the nose and along the columella.

At the end of the operation both nostrils are gently packed with ribbon gauze. This prevents blood collecting between the two layers of mucous membrane and forming a septal haematoma. The packing may be removed on the morning after the operation. As soon as the packing is removed, the nose usually bleeds for a short while and the patient should be warned of this beforehand.

The nose will almost certainly be stuffy for a few days afterwards. The use of 1% ephedrine nose drops and inhalations of menthol and eucalyptus will help to relieve this stuffiness and prevent crusting within the nose.

Nursing management
See Chapter 13.

NASAL POLYPI (Fig. 14/2)

Polypi are bags of waterlogged mucous membrane which arise in the nasal sinuses. The polypi enlarge so that they come to lie within the nose and gradually fill the nasal cavities causing nasal obstruction.

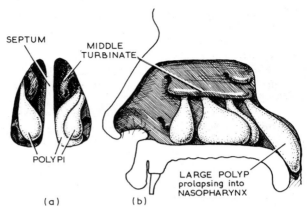

Fig. 14/2 Nasal polypi

The ethmoid sinuses are most commonly affected although polypi may also be found in the maxillary, frontal and sphenoid sinuses. In the majority of cases the exact mechanism by which polypi begin to form is uncertain. In some people *allergy* plays a part while in others polypi are found in association with nasal infections.

The mucous membrane lining the ethmoid sinuses is only loosely attached to the bony walls of the sinuses. For reasons which are not fully understood, watery fluid leaves the blood vessels and accumulates in the mucous membrane which then becomes oedematous and pale. As more and more fluid accumulates, the oedema increases. The waterlogged mucous membrane then begins to sag under the influence of gravity until a polyp has formed. As the polyp increases in size, so the nose becomes more blocked.

Symptoms

Nasal obstruction which is usually bilateral.

Nasal discharge: this is usually clear and watery, but it may be purulent if there is associated infection.

Anosmia (loss of sense of smell).

Bouts of sneezing.

Headaches.

The appearance of a nasal polyp is not unlike that of a skinned grape. Polypi are usually relatively insensitive to touch.

Treatment

There is no effective medical treatment and nasal polypi should be removed surgically using a snare (Fig. 14/3). If there are only a few polypi it may be possible to remove them under local anaesthesia, otherwise a general anaesthetic will be required.

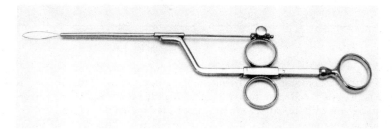

Fig. 14/3 Snare to remove polypi

The wire loop of the snare is manoeuvred around the polyp and slid up around its neck as high as possible. The wire is then tightened and the polyp cut off at its point of attachment. There is often a small amount of bleeding so the nose may be lightly packed with ribbon gauze impregnated with petroleum jelly.

Unfortunately polypi have a tendency to grow again after a variable period of time, and the patient should be warned that further operations may be required. If the polypi recur quickly, and in great numbers, then it may be necessary to carry out further surgery aimed at clearing the ethmoid sinuses more thoroughly. These are the operations of intranasal, transantral, or external ethmoidectomies.

The prescription of low-dose, long-term steroids by mouth may help to keep the nose free of polypi.

Nursing care

See Chapter 13.

CHAPTER FIFTEEN

Malignant Tumours of the Maxillary Sinus: Maxillectomy

The most commonly occurring malignant tumour of the sinuses is a squamous cell carcinoma of the maxillary sinus. More rarely, malignant tumours affect the frontal and the sphenoid sinuses.

Carcinoma of the maxillary sinus arises from the mucosal lining and may be present for a long time before becoming apparent. This is because the interior of the maxillary sinus is a relatively 'silent' area, and, indeed, the tumour may only become apparent after it has breached the bony boundaries of the sinus.

If the tumour spreads *medially* into the nasal cavity it will give rise to a unilateral nasal blockage with bloodstained nasal discharge. If the tumour advances *forward*, the cheek may become swollen and numb as the cutaneous nerves are destroyed. If there is *downward* spread of the growth the hard palate may become swollen or may ulcerate and the teeth may become loosened. If there is *upward* tumour spread the thin bony roof of the antrum can be destroyed, the orbit invaded and the eye displaced. This may give rise to unilateral exophthalmus or diplopia.

Once the tumour has invaded an area of soft tissue with a rich lymphatic supply, it may spread and give rise to cervical lymph node metastases. This is a later phenomenon and carries a poor prognosis. Blood-borne metastases are rare.

Radiographic examination of the sinus will show an opaque antrum on the affected side with erosion of the bony sinus walls.

TREATMENT

A biopsy is essential and can best be obtained by exploring the antrum through a Caldwell-Luc approach (see Fig. 12/2, p. 104). Once the diagnosis has been confirmed treatment usually takes the form of a combination of radiotherapy and surgery.

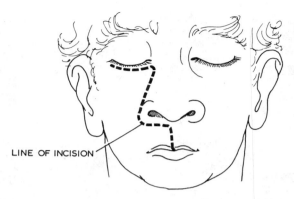

LINE OF INCISION

Fig. 15/1 The incision for a maxillectomy

The surgical operation of choice is a total maxillectomy, though smaller less radical operations may be performed if the growth is small. Figure 15/1 indicates the extent of the incision which may be required. Involvement of the orbit may sometimes be obvious and will require enucleation of the eye. In some instances, however, evidence of orbital involvement only becomes apparent at the time of operation. If there is any uncertainty pre-operatively this fact should be carefully and kindly explained to the patient by the surgeon who should point out, without being overdramatic or frightening the patient, the risk of leaving behind an eye involved by the tumour. Such an eye would soon become blind and painful and would represent residual tumour thereby lessening the chance of cure. *Specific consent* should therefore be obtained for removing the eye at the time of the maxillectomy, if this is necessary.

The majority of patients would be understandably upset by the prospect of losing an eye and may have genuine fears regarding what they imagine to be a very disfiguring procedure perhaps with serious social consequences. They will worry what they are going to look like after the operation, but it should be sympathetically explained to them that nowadays it *is* possible to cover the defect with a realistic prosthesis – Figure 15/2(a) and (b) shows such a prosthesis attached to a spectacle frame.

A nurse should accompany the surgeon while he talks to the patient because it is likely that the patient will have doubts and fears that he is unwilling at first to discuss with the surgeon. He will

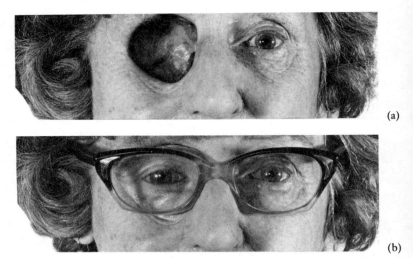

(a)

(b)

Fig. 15/2 (a) *above* Orbital enucleation (b) *below* The defect covered by a prosthesis attached to a spectacle frame

probably welcome the opportunity of sharing his anxieties with a nurse who may then be able to put his mind at rest, or relay the fears to the surgeon who can then talk to the patient again.

The operation
At operation the maxilla on the affected side, together with the eye, if necessary, is removed. Occasionally, a split skin graft may be used to line the cavity. At the same time the patient will be fitted with a dental plate to which an obturator is added to fill the gap left by removal of the maxilla (Fig. 15/3). A member of the oral surgery department will have seen the patient pre-operatively and dental impressions will have been taken to help with the fitting of the dental plate.

The dental obturator is usually held in place by wires, and some days postoperatively the wires are removed and the dental plate taken out so that the cavity can be inspected (this is usually done without an anaesthetic). The plate and obturator will almost certainly need minor adjustments, and ultimately a lightweight plastic obturator will be made which the patient can slip in and out easily for regular cleaning just like an ordinary dental plate.

The maxillectomy cavity itself will need regular cleaning while the patient is in hospital and by the patient himself after discharge from hospital. There is a tendency for mucus to dry and to form soft crusts inside the cavity. These crusts may be gently removed by irrigating the cavity with warm water or a weak solution of sodium bicarbonate, using a 20ml syringe with a soft plastic quill on the end to enable irrigating solution to be gently squirted into the cavity. This may be done over a bowl or at the wash basin.

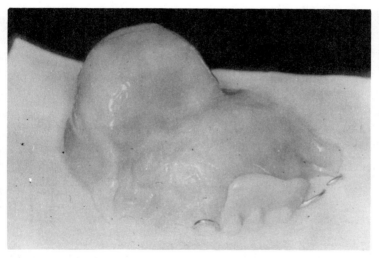

Fig. 15/3 An obturator attached to a dental plate. This patient had some natural teeth (courtesy Professor J.R. Moore)

Follow-up

The exact programme for fitting and adjusting the plate and obturator will depend on the policy of the oral surgery department who will continue to see the patient in the outpatient department after his discharge.

Any patient who has had treatment for a malignant condition needs careful follow-up. In many hospitals there are joint clinics run by radiotherapists and surgeons who will examine patients carefully for any sign of recurrent disease. A patient who has had a maxillectomy is no exception and the patient will be seen regularly so that the maxillectomy cavity may be inspected. The neck will also be carefully palpated for any sign of metastatic lymph node involvement, which might require further radiotherapy or a block dissection (see Chapter 21).

Section Three – The Mouth and Throat

CHAPTER SIXTEEN

Anatomy and Physiology

TEETH (Fig. 16/1)

Everyone has two sets of teeth, the *milk teeth* which appear between the 6th and 24th month of life, and the *permanent dentition* which replace the milk teeth between the ages of 6 and 24 years. Both sets of tooth buds are present at birth.

Teeth are of four types, incisors (I), canine (C), premolars (P) and molars (M). In each quadrant (half of the jaw) they are arranged as follows:

	I	*C*	*P*	*M*
milk teeth	2	1	–	2
permanent teeth	2	1	2	3

This gives a total of 20 milk teeth and 32 permanent teeth.

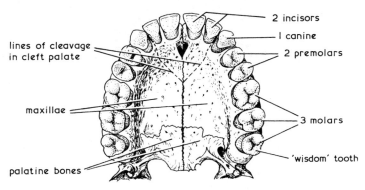

lines of cleavage in cleft palate

2 incisors

I canine

2 premolars

maxillae

3 molars

'wisdom' tooth

palatine bones

Fig. 16/1 Permanent dentition of the upper jaw

The teeth erupt at approximately the following times (there may be individual variations):

MILK TEETH (time in months)

	I	C	P	M
upper jaw	7–8	18	–	12–24
lower jaw	6–9	18	–	12–24

PERMANENT DENTITION (time in years)

	I	C	P	M
upper jaw	7–8	12	9–10	6, 12, 18–24
lower jaw	7–8	12	9–10	6, 12, 18–24

The permanent teeth of the lower jaw tend to erupt slightly earlier than those of the upper jaw.

THE TONGUE (Fig. 16/2)

The tongue is a muscular organ covered by a mucous membrane with a rich sensory nerve supply. The tongue has an important part to play in chewing by keeping the food between the teeth, it also aids in the early part of swallowing by pressing the bolus of food against the hard palate first by the tip and then further back by the dorsum of the tongue.

Sounds produced by the larynx are modified by the lips, tongue

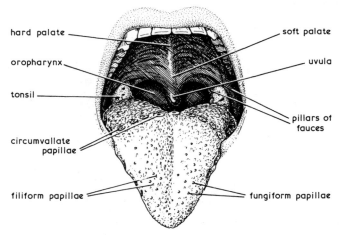

Fig. 16/2 The tongue

and teeth to make the speech sounds. This is the process of articu-
lation.

The tongue is also an important sensory organ, associated with
the sensation of taste.

Both the intrinsic tongue muscles and the larger extrinsic muscles
which connect the tongue to the mandible, hyoid bone, styloid process and hard palate, change the position and shape of the tongue.

Mucous membrane

The mucous membrane on the dorsum of the tongue is rough and
thick and contains many papillae as well as the taste buds. Towards
the back of the tongue the larger vallate papillae can be seen arranged
in the shape of an inverted V, i.e. ∧.

The epithelium covering the floor of the mouth and sides of the
tongue is thin, smooth and shiny.

On the undersurface of the tongue there is a fold of mucous
membrane in the midline. This is called the *frenulum* and at times
may be particularly short and give rise to the condition of tongue-
tie. The submandibular salivary ducts open on to a small papilla on
either side of the frenulum.

Taste

The taste buds of the posterior third of the tongue are supplied by
the glossopharyngeal nerve which also subserves common sensation
in this region. In the anterior two thirds of the tongue the taste buds
are supplied by the chorda tympani fibres in the lingual nerve.

SUBMANDIBULAR SALIVARY GLANDS (Fig. 16/3)

There are two submandibular salivary glands one on each side beneath the floor of the mouth adjacent to the mandible. Sometimes,
little stones form either in the gland or in the main duct. These
stones prevent the drainage of saliva from the gland and cause the
gland to become painfully swollen. The condition may be relieved
by removing the stone, but if the gland itself is damaged it may have
to be removed through an incision in the neck below the mandible.

PAROTID SALIVARY GLANDS (Fig. 16/3)

These are the largest of the salivary glands. On each side, the gland

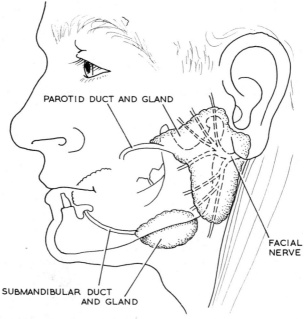

PAROTID DUCT AND GLAND

FACIAL
NERVE

SUBMANDIBULAR DUCT
AND GLAND

Fig. 16/3 The submandibular and parotid salivary glands, also showing the relationship of the facial nerve

occupies the space between the posterior edge of the ramus of the mandible in front, and the external auditory canal and mastoid process behind.

The facial nerve which supplies all the muscles of facial expression runs through the centre of the gland after leaving the skull just deep to the mastoid process.

The parotid glands become swollen and painful in mumps. Stones may occur in the parotid duct but these are much less common than in the submandibular salivary duct.

PALATE (Fig. 16/2)

The roof of the mouth is formed by the palate. Anteriorly, the hard palate is bony, while posteriorly the soft palate is formed by muscles covered by mucous membrane. The free margin of the soft palate is enlongated to form the uvula.

On swallowing and on phonation, the soft palate is elevated by muscles and comes to lie against the posterior wall of the pharynx, forming a seal to prevent liquids and solids entering the nose, or air escaping through the nose, respectively.

The small muscles of the soft palate are attached to the opening of the Eustachian tube so that each time a person swallows the Eustachian tube opens, allowing air into the tube and so into the middle ear.

THE TONSILS (Figs. 16/4 and 16/5)

Each palatine tonsil is a collection of lymphoid tissue situated on each side of the posterior part of the oral cavity. The entrance to the pharynx is guarded by an archway called the *fauces*. The roof of the arch corresponds to the soft palate while on each side the tonsil sits between an anterior and a posterior faucial pillar (see Fig. 16/2). These pillars contain muscles which are covered by mucous membrane which is then draped over the free surface of the tonsil. The surface of each tonsil is pitted by tonsillar crypts. The deepest aspect of each tonsil lies against a sheet of muscles, the superior constrictor muscle of the pharynx, to which the capsule of the tonsil is attached only by connective tissue and some blood vessels.

At the base of each tonsil the lymphoid tissue is continuous with a collection of lymphoid tissue at the base of the tongue known as the lingual tonsil. The palatine tonsils, the lingual tonsil and the adenoid pad form a ring of lymphoid tissue which is called

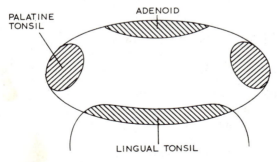

Fig. 16/4 Waldeyer's ring of lymphoid tissue

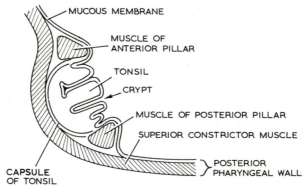

Fig. 16/5 Cross-section through the palatine tonsil

Waldeyer's ring. It encircles the entrance of the air and food passages (Fig. 16/4).

THE PHARYNX (Fig. 16/6)

The pharynx is a muscular tube which starts at the base of the skull and ends at the point where the pharynx joins the oesophagus, at the level of the body of the sixth cervical vertebra. The pharynx is divided into three parts: the nasopharynx, behind the nose; the oropharynx, behind the mouth; and the laryngopharynx, behind the larynx.

The oropharynx forms a common entrance to both the air and food passages.

The pharynx is composed of three main muscles known as constrictor muscles, called superior, middle and inferior from above downward. Each of these muscles is arranged so that it fits into the one below it, like a stack of paper cups (see Fig. 16/9a).

The muscles are attached from above downward to the base of the skull, the mandible, the hyoid bone and to the thyroid and the cricoid cartilages of the larynx. The fibres of each muscle fan out as they pass backward and then meet in the midline to form a fibrous raphe which runs from the skull downward to merge with the fibrous covering of the oesophagus.

Nerve supply to the pharynx (Fig. 16/7)

The motor supply is chiefly from the pharyngeal branches of the

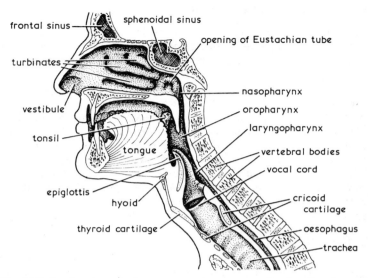

Fig. 16/6 Section through the upper respiratory tract showing the pharynx and its relations

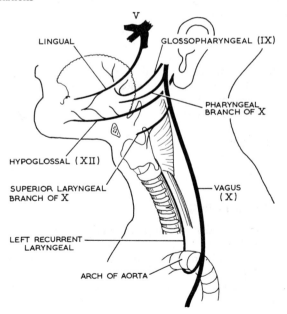

Fig. 16/7 The nerve supply to the pharynx, also showing the course of the vagus (Xth cranial) nerve

vagus nerve (Xth cranial). Smaller contributions are made from the glossopharyngeal nerve (IXth cranial) and the trigeminal nerve (Vth cranial). The main sensory nerves are the glossopharyngeal and vagus nerves.

Swallowing

As food is taken into the mouth it is chewed and then formed into a *bolus* by the action of the jaw and tongue. The bolus is then transferred towards the back of the tongue by elevating the tip against the roof of the mouth and squeezing the bolus backward. The small muscles of the palate pull the soft palate upward and backward against the posterior pharyngeal wall and close off the nasopharynx and nose, so preventing regurgitation. The bolus is then pushed into the oropharynx as the muscles of the faucial pillars contract at the base of the tongue and the hyoid bone is lifted by the action of further muscles.

The larynx is pulled upward and as it does so, the epiglottis flips backward to cover the laryngeal inlet which is then further closed by the sphincter action of the muscles in the ary-epiglottic folds.

The bolus of food slides over the smooth surface of the epiglottis and is then carried on by successive contractions of the superior, middle and inferior constrictors respectively, into the oesophagus. Once in the oesophagus, the bolus is passed downward by rhythmic contractions of the muscular wall, called peristaltic waves.

After the bolus has been passed beyond the laryngeal opening the muscles relax and the larynx is pulled down to its original position by the elastic recoil of the trachea. The soft palate falls and the laryngeal sphincter relaxes so that air can be taken in once more without fear of inhalation of food.

The early stages of swallowing are under voluntary control but as the muscles of the pharynx and oesophagus take over, the movements become involuntary.

CAROTID ARTERIES (Fig. 16/8)

These are the main arteries supplying blood to the head and neck. On the right side the common carotid artery arises from the brachio-cephalic artery, while on the left side it arises direct from the arch of the aorta. The common carotid arteries enter the root of the neck behind the sternoclavicular joints and ascend, under cover of the sternomastoid muscles, to the level of the upper border of the thyroid

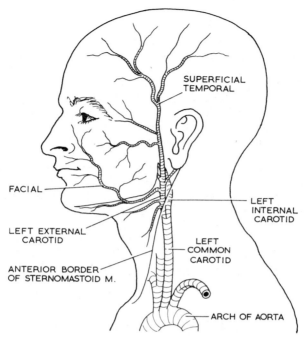

Fig. 16/8 The carotid arteries

cartilage. At this point each common carotid artery divides into an internal and external carotid artery.

The internal carotid artery continues upward and gives off no branches at all until it enters the base of the skull. *The external carotid artery* has many branches which send blood to supply the larynx, pharynx, thyroid gland, tongue, face and scalp while some of the terminal branches supply the nose and sinuses.

The main route for venous drainage is the internal jugular vein which runs vertically, alongside the carotid arteries.

Accompanying these major blood vessels, tucked behind the internal jugular vein, the vagus (Xth cranial nerve) travels through the neck.

THE LARYNX (Fig. 16/9)

The larynx is the specialised upper end of the trachea and separates the pharynx from the trachea and the lungs. The larynx lies in front of the lowermost part of the pharynx and the trachea lies anterior to the oesophagus (Fig. 16/9a).

The larynx is composed of a series of cartilaginous pieces linked together by joints which are then moved by small muscles. The whole is lined by mucous membrane.

The two flat *thyroid cartilages* are hinged anteriorly like the pages of a book and sit on top of a complete ring of cartilage, the *cricoid*. This is shaped rather like a signet ring with the flat vertical plate at the back and a horizontal ring anteriorly. The anterior edge of the thyroid cartilage is easily felt in the neck as the Adam's apple, and below this the anterior part of the cricoid ring may be felt as a smooth bump. On top of the vertical plate of the cricoid are a pair of pyramid-shaped *arytenoid cartilages* which articulate with the cricoid by means of small synovial joints (Fig. 16/9b). The remaining laryngeal cartilage, the *epiglottis*, is leaf-shaped and flexible and is

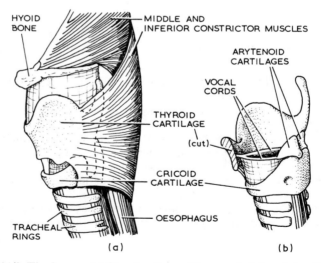

Fig. 16/9 The larynx. (a) Showing the cartilages and their relationship to the muscles of the pharynx; (b) Showing the position of the vocal cords

attached below to the point at which the thyroid cartilages come together anteriorly.

From each arytenoid cartilage a vocal cord passes forward to meet the other vocal cord at the front of the larynx. The point at which the two vocal cords come together is known as the *anterior commissure* and this lies immediately below the point of attachment of the epiglottic cartilage, just behind the laryngeal prominence (Adam's apple).

Movement of the arytenoid cartilages is brought about by the small intrinsic muscles of the larynx which also cause the thyroid cartilages to move upon the cricoid. This results in movement of the vocal cords during phonation, respiration and swallowing.

All the intrinsic muscles of the larynx are supplied by the recurrent laryngeal nerve, a branch of the vagus nerve. The exception to this is the cricothyroid muscle which is supplied by the external branch of the superior laryngeal nerve.

Injury or disease affecting either of the recurrent laryngeal nerves will result in paralysis of the vocal cord and subsequent hoarseness.

The larynx is lined with sensitive mucous membrane. The fold of mucous membrane draped between the arytenoid and the epiglottis is known as the ary-epiglottic fold, and contains the ary-epiglottic muscle.

The most important function of the larynx is to act as a sphincter to prevent aspiration of food and drink from the pharynx into the trachea and lungs. During swallowing, the larynx rises to the level of the back of the tongue. The flexible epiglottic cartilage is flipped backward to cover the laryngeal opening like a lid and is then pulled tightly down by the ary-epiglottic muscles which contract further and narrow the laryngeal opening. The vocal cords come together and so act as a third line of defence. Any food or drink which comes into contact with the sensitive lining of the larynx initiates the cough reflex which then expels the material.

THE TRACHEA (Fig. 16/10)

The trachea is the tube which conveys air from the larynx to the lungs. The trachea is D-shaped in cross-section and is kept open by C-shaped cartilages known as 'rings'. The posterior wall of the trachea is devoid of cartilage and is comprised of fibrous tissue in which there are some smooth muscle fibres.

Immediately behind the trachea lies the oesophagus. The thyroid gland lies astride the trachea, shaped like a butterfly, and the isthmus

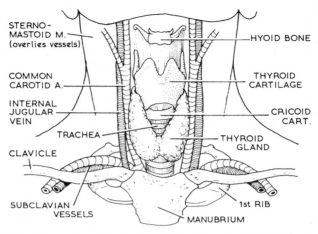

STERNO-
MASTOID M.
(overlies vessels)

HYOID BONE

COMMON
CAROTID A.

THYROID
CARTILAGE

INTERNAL
JUGULAR
VEIN

CRICOID
CART.

TRACHEA

THYROID
GLAND

CLAVICLE

SUBCLAVIAN
VESSELS

1st RIB

MANUBRIUM

Fig. 16/10 The trachea, showing its relationship to the thyroid gland

of the gland usually covers the 2nd, 3rd or 4th rings. At the level of
the manubriosternal joint, the trachea divides into the right and left
main bronchi which enter the lungs.

THE LYMPHATIC DRAINAGE OF THE
HEAD AND NECK (Fig. 16/11)

All the structures of the head and neck with the exception of the
bone, cartilage and the central nervous system, are richly supplied
with small, thin-walled lymph vessels.

Lymph from these vessels drains into lymph nodes. From these
nodes, further vessels transport the lymph to other lymph nodes
before it is collected into lymph trunks. On the left side, these drain
into the *thoracic duct*. On the right side, the lymph either drains into
the right lymph duct or directly into the great veins at the junction
of the subclavian and internal jugular veins.

Lymph nodes

These are arranged into various groups. The *deep cervical group* lie
vertically in a line reaching from the base of the skull to the root of
the neck, and for the most part, lie on the carotid sheath alongside
the internal jugular vein, deep to the sternomastoid muscle.

Most of the lymph that reaches the deep cervical chain has already

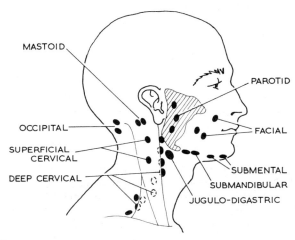

Fig. 16/11 The lymphatic drainage of the head and neck

filtered through other nodes that are arranged in two circles – an outer and an inner circle.

The *outer circle* is made up of superficial nodes from occiput to chin, while the *inner circle* lies within it and surrounds the upper air and food passages.

Many of the nodes in the neck may be subdivided into smaller groups and some individual nodes are named. The most easily palpable and most commonly enlarged node is a member of the deep cervical chain, and lies between the angle of the mandible and the anterior border of the mandible. It is known as the *jugulo-digastric node*, and, among other structures, drains the tonsil.

CHAPTER SEVENTEEN

Stridor

Stridor is an abnormal noise arising from the lower respiratory tract. It is an important symptom because it indicates that there is an obstruction to the passage of air through the larynx, trachea or main bronchi which may have to be relieved by the introduction of an endotracheal tube or the making of a tracheostomy.

By listening carefully to the stridor it should be possible to determine in which phase of the respiratory cycle the stridor occurs and this helps to decide at which site the obstruction has occurred.

Inspiratory stridor: This often has a 'crowing' quality and may be called *croup*. The cause is usually in the larynx.

Expiratory stridor: This is usually due to bronchial obstruction and is referred to as *'wheezing'*.

Two-way stridor: This occurs in both phases of respiration and usually signifies partial obstruction in the trachea.

In an adult, inspiratory stridor may be caused by laryngeal carcinoma and there may be accompanying symptoms of hoarseness, dyspnoea, or cough. Stridor may also arise following thyroid surgery if the recurrent laryngeal nerves are damaged and there is impaired movement of the vocal cords.

STRIDOR IN CHILDHOOD

This always requires prompt investigation to establish the cause. Once the cause is known precisely then the appropriate treatment may be started. As in every condition accurate diagnosis depends on the history, examination, and special investigations.

History
The taking of a history needs to take account of the following: How

long has the noise been present? If it started suddenly, what was the child doing at the time the noise started? If he was eating it is possible that something may have been inhaled. If the noise has been present since birth are there any associated symptoms such as feeding difficulties, cough, recurrent chest infections, or an abnormal cry?

Examination

By listening to the child's breathing, and physically examining the chest the doctor can determine where in the respiratory cycle the stridor occurs (see above). Is the noise affected by changes in posture? If the noise disappears it may arise from one of the surrounding structures rather than coming from the airway itself.

Are there any signs of respiratory obstruction such as intercostal recession?

Investigation

Unless the child's condition is giving rise to grave concern and some intervention to protect the child's airway is anticipated, a plain radiograph of the chest and neck should be taken. A barium swallow should also be requested as this will demonstrate any inco-ordination or spill-over into the trachea and will also show if there is anything pressing on the trachea such as an abnormal blood vessel in the mediastinum.

Because it is essential to make a definite diagnosis the child should be examined by an otolaryngologist who is familiar which paediatric endoscopy, working with an experienced paediatric anaesthetist. It is necessary to perform a microlaryngoscopy and bronchoscopy.

Treatment

This depends on the diagnosis but the surgeon will do whatever is necessary to preserve the patient's airway and this may involve a tracheostomy (see Chapter 18). Endoscopic examination must be followed by a period of careful supervision with oxygen and humidification on hand to assist breathing. Suction must always be available.

While it is inappropriate in this book to give an account of the many conditions which give rise to stridor in childhood and their treatment, we may discuss the more common causes.

LARYNGOMALACIA (CONGENITAL LARYNGEAL STRIDOR)

In simple terms this may be thought of as a 'floppy larynx', and the parts of the larynx just above the level of the vocal cords are sucked in during inspiration. The condition tends to improve gradually as the child grows older but he may be four or five before the noise goes altogether. The stridor may worsen with a respiratory tract infection and the parents should be told to bring the child into hospital for observation and treatment if this occurs.

SUBGLOTTIC STENOSIS

This is a narrowing of the airway just below the vocal cords. It may be congenital but sometimes it is seen in babies born prematurely who require artificial ventilation. The narrowing may occur as a result of damage caused by the presence of an endotracheal tube for a long time. Mild cases may require nothing more than prompt treatment of respiratory tract infections when the stridor may worsen (croup). Severe cases may require tracheostomy and later, when the child is two or more years of age, an operation may be required to correct the narrowing.

VOCAL CORD PALSY

This may affect one or both vocal cords and sometimes is the result of birth trauma or raised intracranial pressure. Often the cause is unknown. In cases where there is severe respiratory obstruction a tracheostomy may be required. Recovery may occur spontaneously, so repeated examinations of the larynx are necessary to monitor progress.

Stridor presenting in otherwise healthy children may be due to:
1. Acute inflammation of the larynx or trachea.
2. An inhaled foreign body.
3. A benign laryngeal tumour.
Urgent hospital admission is required for diagnosis and treatment.

ACUTE INFLAMMATION

In the United Kingdom the most common acute inflammatory conditions causing stridor and respiratory obstruction are acute epiglottis and acute laryngo-tracheo-bronchitis.

In some parts of the world diphtheria still exists as the most common and fatal cause of croup.

In all these conditions the onset and progression of symptoms may be very rapid and fatal so prompt treatment is very necessary. The most important factors in management are:

(a) Protection of the airway. Endotracheal intubation or tracheostomy may be needed.
(b) Humidification of air to loosen the secretions and prevent crusting.
(c) Identification and treatment of the infecting organism with antibiotics.
(d) Treatment of the inflammatory swelling with steroids.

INHALED FOREIGN BODIES

These must be removed as soon as possible. This is especially important in the case of vegetable foreign bodies which rapidly give rise to serious pneumonia.

BENIGN LARYNGEAL TUMOURS

The most common are haemangiomata which may be accompanied by haemangiomata elsewhere on the body, and papillomata. The latter may be single or multiple and require regular removal as there is a marked tendency for these warty tumours to recur. If respiratory obstruction is severe a preliminary tracheostomy may be necessary.

NURSING CARE OF CHILD WITH CROUP OR EPIGLOTTITIS

1. *Isolation:* In some units it is the policy to isolate these children and so minimise the risk of infecting others.
2. *Observation:* The pulse, respiratory rate, quality of breathing, colour and general appearance should be noted hourly for signs of increased respiratory difficulty. The temperature should be recorded 1-4-hourly.

   In addition to these specific observations the child should be placed in such a position in the ward where he can be clearly seen *at all times* so that any worsening of the clinical condition can be immediately seen.

3. *Humidified atmosphere:* There should be either a unit blowing steam into the room or over the patient or via a humidity tent. The latter is particularly helpful if oxygen is also required. The nurse should always remember that tents may be very frightening for children and may exacerbate their condition. Continued reassurance is therefore essential.

4. If the patient's colour is poor, oxygen may be required and the prescribed amount should be monitored.

5. If the child is restless this may be due to anoxia and the treatment should be with oxygen and *not* with sedation.

6. *Position:* The child is usually more comfortable supported by pillows in a semi-sitting position.

7. The child should wear loose clothing.

8. The child should be allowed small, frequent drinks, and the nurse must make sure he is able to swallow.

9. If the throat is sore, analgesia in the form of paracetamol or soluble aspirin may help.

10. A calm, confident atmosphere is most important. The child will require much reassurance and adequate rest must be ensured.

11. Throat swabs should not be taken unless an experienced doctor is present. Gagging may produce laryngeal spasm.

12. If severe respiratory distress occurs, tracheostomy or endotracheal intubation may be necessary. Therefore an emergency resuscitation trolley *must* be available at all times.

CHAPTER EIGHTEEN

Tracheostomy

Tracheostomy is the operation to make an opening into the trachea through the skin at the front of the neck.

INDICATIONS

1. To relieve obstruction in the upper airway.
2. To protect the lungs against inhalation of blood or secretions.
3. To provide a means of administering long-term artificial ventilation.

Obstruction

Respiratory obstruction may occur at any anatomical level down as far as the trachea. Causes include:

1. Congenital, e.g. a congenital subglottic stenosis occurring in infants and young children.
2. Infection, e.g. acute epiglottitis.
3. Allergic, e.g. angioneurotic oedema affecting the larynx.
4. Accidental, e.g. an inhaled foreign body impacted in the larynx.
5. Neurological, e.g. bilateral vocal cord palsy resulting from damage to the recurrent laryngeal nerves during thyroid surgery.
6. Tumours: *Benign*, e.g. multiple papillomata of the larynx; *Malignant*, e.g. carcinoma of the larynx.

Some patients who are having radiotherapy for carcinoma of the larynx may develop considerable oedema of the larynx requiring a temporary tracheostomy.

Inhalation

If major surgery is to be performed on the tongue, floor of the mouth or lower jaw, such as the excision of a tumour, and there is a risk of heavy bleeding both during and after the operation, it is safer to perform a preliminary tracheostomy. This will protect the airway against inhalation of blood or secretions.

Respiratory failure
Patients with respiratory failure occurring after a drug overdose, following major surgery, particularly cardiothoracic or major trauma may require artificial ventilation.

Artificial ventilation can usually be administered by an endo-tracheal tube passed through the nose or mouth into the larynx and upper trachea. (This is usually done by an anaesthetist.) The pressure exerted on the delicate mucosal lining of the larynx and trachea by the inflated cuff of the tube will eventually damage the mucosa and the underlying cartilage. This could result in scarring and permanent narrowing of the airway. If artificial ventilation has to be maintained for more than five to seven days, a tracheostomy should be performed.

Such a tracheostomy is usually *temporary* and may be required only for a day or so, or may need to be retained for weeks or months. In the majority of cases, however, the tracheostomy will eventually be reversed.

If the tracheostomy has been done for carcinoma of the larynx and is then followed by a laryngectomy the tracheostomy will be converted to an end-tracheostomy by bringing the cut end of the trachea out on to the skin.

The operation (Figs. 18/1 and 18/2)
In an emergency when it is not possible to give the patient a general anaesthetic the operation may be performed under local anaesthetic. It is far better, however, to anticipate the need for a tracheostomy and to carry out the operation as a planned procedure, with a general anaesthetic, in a fully equipped operating theatre with good lighting and the correct instruments. Figure 18/2 shows a standard pack of instruments for performing a tracheostomy.

The patient is anaesthetised and placed on the operating table with a sandbag under the shoulders. This extends the neck and makes the larynx more prominent. The skin is cleaned and towels are applied. An infiltration of local anaesthetic, e.g. lignocaine 0.5%, and adrenaline 1 in 200 000 into the skin will reduce the amount of bleeding from the skin and subcutaneous tissues.

A horizontal incision is made approximately midway between the cricoid cartilage and the suprasternal notch. Small bleeding points

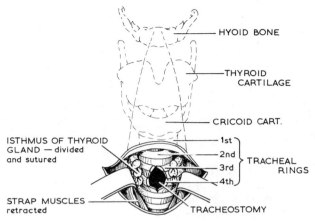

Fig. 18/1 Tracheostomy

are sealed with diathermy and the larger vessels are tied with catgut. The thin muscles which run vertically in the neck in front of the larynx and trachea (strap muscles) are separated in the midline and retracted laterally. This exposes the isthmus of the thyroid gland which sits in front of the trachea. The isthmus may have to be divided between clips, and the cut edges of the thyroid gland are transfixed with a suture to prevent bleeding. It should be possible now to identify the cricoid cartilage and the upper tracheal rings.

An opening is made into the front wall of the trachea centred on the 3rd or 4th tracheal ring and a cuffed tracheostomy tube of the appropriate size is carefully passed into the trachea. The anaesthetist connects the supply of anaesthetic gases to the tracheostomy tube and removes the endotracheal tube. The cuff on the tube is gently inflated until there is an airtight seal between it and the wall of the trachea.

After ensuring that bleeding has ceased, silk sutures are placed loosely in the skin to prevent the wound from gaping.

The tube is held in place by tapes tied securely round the neck with three *knots*. **Never** use bows as they may become accidentally undone, allowing the tube to slip out and be impossible to replace. A sterile non–adherent dressing is placed under the tube next to the skin.

The cuff on the tube should be deflated as soon as possible because the pressure exerted on the tracheal mucosa by the cuff interferes

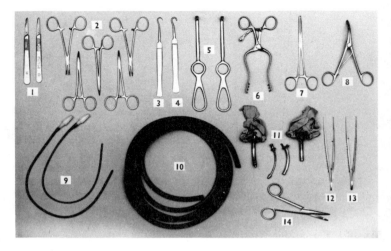

Fig. 18/2 A standard tracheostomy pack.
1. 2 Bard Parker handles No. 3 and 7 with No. 15 blades; 2. 5 Curved mosquito artery clips; 3. 1 Sharp single hook; 4. 1 Blunt single hook; 5. 2 Langenbeck's retractors; 6. 2 RNTNE retractors; 7. 1 Alliss tissue forceps; 8. 1 Tracheal dilator; 9. 2 Jacques catheters 10 and 12 FG; 10. Length of suction tubing; 11. 2 sets of Jackson's tracheostomy tubes size 24 FG (other sizes may be required); 12. 1 Silcock toothed forceps; 13. 1 Silcock non-toothed forceps; 14. 1 May's curved scissors

with the flow of blood through the mucosal vessels. If the blood supply is cut off the tracheal mucosa will ulcerate and die, exposing the underlying tracheal cartilage. The unprotected cartilage will then also necrose and become infected. The result will be scarring and contraction with the formation of a stenosis at the site of the tracheostomy tube cuff. The nurse must check that the cuff is only inflated to the minimum pressure necessary to produce a seal and that it is periodically deflated.

NURSING MANAGEMENT

Tracheostomy is usually an emergency procedure performed because of difficulty with breathing; oxygen and humidification must be available immediately.

The patient should be constantly 'specialed' by a nurse who will need to spend much time reassuring both the patient and his relatives. If there is any deterioration in breathing the medical staff should be notified immediately.

Postoperative
Unless there are intensive-care facilities the patient will probably be nursed in a side room which should be prepared with all the equipment required to care for him. This will include:
1. An electrically operated humidifier. (This must be checked to make sure it is running properly before the patient returns from theatre.)
2. Oxygen. If piped oxygen is unavailable, cylinders will be used and a spare cylinder must always be available. Oxygen is usually given via the humidifier.
3. A tray containing the following:
   Tracheal dilators
   A selection of plastic tracheostomy tubes
   Suction catheters (size 12 is average)
   Sterile water
   A foil bowl
   A box of disposable gloves
   A large bag for disposing of catheters and gloves
   Gauze squares or lyofoam squares to be put round the tracheostomy tube
   A syringe for inflating and deflating the cuff of the tracheostomy tube
   KY jelly for lubricating the catheter
   Rogers crystal spray – filled with normal saline
4. Suction equipment
5. Writing equipment as the patient is unable to talk
6. An infusion stand
7. A bell so that the patient can ring for help – it is desirable that a nurse remains with a patient who has had a tracheostomy.

On return from theatre the patient is usually sitting upright to enable easier breathing. A cuffed plastic tracheostomy tube will be in position – the cuff prevents secretions, such as blood oozing from the suture line, trickling down the trachea and into the lungs. An intravenous infusion will usually be in position. The patient should be made comfortable with the head and neck supported. The blood pressure and pulse should be monitored and regular recordings made.

SUCTION CARE

This is an aseptic procedure to avoid introducing infection. The nurse should check that all the equipment that she will need is at hand. Then she washes and dries her hands and puts on disposable gloves. A catheter is fixed to the Y-connection of the suction tubing and the suction turned on. The nurse takes an empty syringe and withdraws the air from the cuffed tracheostomy tube noting the amount withdrawn. A small amount of normal saline from the crystal spray is introduced into the tracheostomy tube prior to suction; this helps to prevent crusting within the tube.

The catheter is withdrawn from its sterile cover taking care that the tip of the catheter does not touch anything. It is introduced into the tracheostomy tube so that the tip of the catheter reaches just beyond the distal end of the tracheostomy tube; suction is applied by putting a finger over the free end of the Y-connection and the catheter twisted round and withdrawn (this should be done fairly briskly and should not cause trauma to the trachea wall). The used catheter is then disposed of by wrapping it round one hand and then pulling the glove off so that the catheter remains inside. If further suction is needed the procedure is repeated using a clean catheter and gloves.

The suction tubing is flushed through with a solution of sodium bicarbonate before turning off the suction. The cuff is then re-inflated with the same amount of air that was withdrawn at the start of the procedure.

The patient may find this procedure uncomfortable, causing him to cough while it is being done; the nurse will have to reassure him constantly. The fact that a tracheostomy precludes talking adds to a patient's apprehension. Questions should be so worded that an answer can be indicated by nodding or shaking the head: writing materials must be provided – a Magic-writer is very useful for it can be cleaned each time it is used. The nurse must talk to the patient whenever she is with him.

Immediately postoperatively, hourly suction and spraying is sufficient unless there are excessive secretions.

Analgesics should be given regularly for pain relief. If the surgeon is satisfied, and the patient conscious and co-operative, oral fluids may commence the following morning. If the patient is unable to swallow, a nasogastric tube will have been passed in theatre. Mouth care needs to be carried out regularly until the fluid intake is sufficient. The patient should be mobilised within his limitations as soon as possible. If he is unconscious, passive movements of all limbs will be required. Particular care is required for the pressure areas.

Regular physiotherapy in the form of breathing exercises and vibrations and shakings to the chest wall will help to clear secretions. The nurse should carry out suction while the physiotherapist vibrates the chest.

CHANGING THE TUBE

It is advisable to leave the first change of tube for three or four days after the original operation; by then a track will have formed and the tube will be easier to replace. If the tube becomes crusted it will need to be replaced sooner.

If the patient is unconscious or his breathing is being maintained on a ventilator a cuffed tube will be re-inserted. If the patient is to have radiotherapy an uncuffed plastic tube should be used but otherwise a silver tube with a valved speaking attachment may be inserted.

Procedure

1. The new tracheostomy tube should be taken out of its package and checked that it is the correct size. If it is a silver tube all the parts should be seen to fit together snugly.
2. The trachea is sucked out using aseptic precautions.
3. The tapes are cut and all neck dressings removed.
4. The new tracheostomy tube is picked up with the right hand.
5. Using the left hand the old tube is removed and immediately the new tube (held in the right hand) is inserted through the same opening. This usually promotes a bout of coughing and the secretions may need to be sucked out, keeping one hand on the tube to make sure that it is not coughed out. The neck skin is cleaned and the tapes are securely tied.

TRACHEOSTOMY TUBES (Fig. 18/3)

All tracheostomy tubes consist of a curved tube which passes into the trachea, and a flange which lies against the skin of the neck to which tapes are attached to maintain the tube firmly in place. The various tubes differ slightly in design and may be made of different materials such as stainless steel, silver, plastics, rubber. The tube chosen for an individual patient will depend on the circumstances of the particular case. All the tubes are available in a variety of sizes.

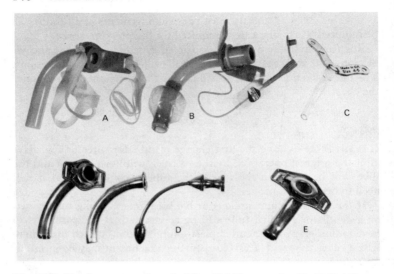

Fig. 18/3 Tracheostomy tubes. A. Uncuffed Portex tube; B. Cuffed Portex tube; C. Paediatric tube; D. Negus silver tube showing a plain outer and inner tube, a valved inner tube and an introducer; E. Laryngectomy tube

Cuffed plastic tube (Fig. 18/3B)

Once the tube is in position in the trachea the cuff may be inflated to produce an airtight seal. This type of tube is particularly useful for patients receiving artificial ventilation or as the first tube inserted following a tracheostomy when the cuff may be inflated to prevent aspiration of blood from the wound into the trachea and lungs. The cuff must not be over-inflated otherwise the tracheal wall may be damaged resulting in tracheal stenosis; nowadays high-volume/low-pressure cuffs minimise this occurrence.

All plastic tubes are disposable and need to be changed regularly as they become crusted and tend to become blocked.

Uncuffed plastic tubes (Fig. 18/3A)

When there is no longer a risk of the wound bleeding into the trachea the cuffed tube may be replaced by an uncuffed one. Such a tube is also used for patients who have to have a tracheostomy while undergoing a course of radiotherapy for laryngeal carcinoma.

Paediatric tracheostomy tube – plastic (Fig. 18/3C)
Because of the relatively smaller size of a child's trachea, paediatric tracheostomy tubes are not cuffed because the cuff would take up too much room and would not allow a sufficiently large tube for breathing.

Silver tracheostomy tube (Fig. 18/3D)
This tube consists of an outer tube, an introducer and an inner tube. Silver tubes are usually easy for the patient to manage and therefore suitable for the patient with a long-term tracheostomy. They are not suitable for patients undergoing radiotherapy to the neck because the metal tube disperses the beam of radiotherapy.

While the outer tube may be left in place for up to one week the inner tube must be removed regularly for cleaning. The inner tube is slightly longer than the outer tube and crusts tend to collect on the end of the inner tube: if they are not removed the tube will become blocked and the patient will not have a patent airway. The inner tube may be fitted with a small flap valve. This allows the patient to inspire normally, but on expiration the flap valve shuts and the air is directed upward towards the vocal cords, thus allowing the patient to talk. Such a tube is called a *speaking tube*.

Laryngectomy tube (Fig. 18/3E)
A laryngectomy tube has a slightly different shape to a conventional tracheostomy tube and is thus more suited for patients who have a permanent end-tracheostome. These tubes are usually made of silver, although some may be made of a plastic material.

CHAPTER NINETEEN

Throat surgery: Tonsillectomy: Adenoidectomy

Throat operations may conveniently be divided into two groups depending on the method of approach, internal or external.

INTERNAL APPROACH

This approach concerns those operations which require access to the upper air or food passages through the open mouth. It includes endoscopic examination. The majority of such operations are carried out with the patient lying supine on the operating table with the surgeon standing or sitting at the head of the table (Fig. 19/1).

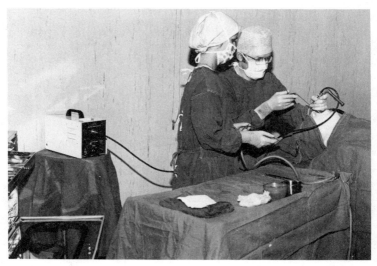

Fig. 19/1 Endoscopy examination

For certain operations, such as tonsillectomy, the mouth is held open by a gag and, if bleeding is anticipated, the patient's shoulders are supported on a small sandbag. This means that blood will collect in the pharynx at a lower level than the larynx and so will not be aspirated into the lungs.

The key to safety and success in operations done through the open mouth is co-operation and understanding between surgeon and anaesthetist. At all times the anaesthetist must have access to the patient's airway, yet he must be able to position his tubes and connections in such a way as to allow the surgeon the best possible access to operate safely. It is their joint responsibility to ensure that no blood or secretions enter the larynx, but while the surgeon is actually operating the greater responsibility rests with the surgeon. Any blood or secretions in the pharynx are removed by suction.

Procedures to inspect the inside of one of the body orifices are known as endoscopies. The instruments used and the procedure take their names from the part to be examined – thus a laryngoscope is used for the larynx and the operation is called a laryngoscopy. The majority of these instruments (endoscopes) are rigid metal tubes with a handle for holding and a light, usually at the proximal end so that the structures can be visualised. In recent years there has been

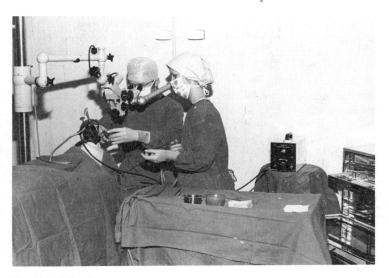

Fig. 19/2 Microlaryngoscopy

considerable improvement in light sources and in the design of lenses so that now there is an increasing tendency to perform endoscopies using telescopes which give a highly illuminated, magnified view through a narrower instrument. Flexible, fibre-optic instruments are also used.

When examining the larynx it is possible to use the operating microscope to look down the laryngoscope. Under this magnification, surgery to the vocal cords may be carried out with more precision to give a better functional result. The technique is called micro-laryngoscopy (Fig. 19/2).

A biopsy of abnormal tissue seen at endoscopy can be carried out with specially designed forceps.

EXTERNAL APPROACH

By implication this indicates the need to make an incision or incisions through the skin of the neck to allow exposure of those parts requiring surgery.

Operations such as total laryngectomy and removal of malignant lymph nodes will be carried out using one or more skin incisions. Where it is necessary to protect the lungs from blood or secretions after the operation or where part of the upper airway, such as the larynx, is removed, the patient will be given a tracheostomy (see Chapter 18). If swallowing is likely to be difficult or impossible, a nasogastric tube will be passed to enable the patient to be fed.

Before finally closing the incision, one or more drains will be inserted into the wound (see Fig. 20/2, p. 166). This prevents the accumulation of blood and fluid under the incision or skin flaps. The drains may consist of corrugated plastic or may be of rubber or plastic tubing which can be attached to suction. Once any drainage has ceased the drains are removed, usually after 24–48 hours.

TONSILLECTOMY

In the child the tonsils play an important part in the development of resistance to infection. Acute infections of the tonsils are not infrequent in children and are to be expected as part of the process of normal development.

Indications for tonsillectomy

IN THE CHILD

1. Repeated attacks of true acute tonsillitis, particularly if associated with otitis media and deafness. The child may be losing considerable time from school and be failing to gain weight.
2. Respiratory obstruction, if the tonsils are very large (this is not common).
3. After a quinsy (peritonsillar abscess). A quinsy rarely occurs in a child but it is an indication for tonsillectomy after an interval of five to six weeks. Further attacks of quinsy might result in the spread of infection through the fascial planes of the neck and this must be avoided since it could lead to a fatal mediastinitis.

IN THE ADULT

1. Recurrent attacks of acute tonsillitis.
2. Following quinsy.
3. For histology. If there is enlargement of one tonsil only, or progressive ulceration of one tonsil, the tonsil should be removed and examined histologically in case the tonsil has undergone malignant change.

Acute tonsillitis

Probably the majority of attacks are due to a virus, and antibiotics are of no real value. Tonsillitis is a self-limiting disease which lasts about six days and is accompanied by pyrexia and dysphagia.

If the history is one of repeated sore throats occurring every day for weeks or months, often worse in the morning, then the diagnosis is more likely to be chronic pharyngitis due to dental sepsis, infection in the nose or sinuses, or breathing through the mouth. There is no pyrexia or dysphagia. Tonsillectomy is not indicated.

Quinsy (Fig. 19/3)

This is the term used to describe a collection of pus around the tonsil (peritonsillar abscess). The patient is usually a young adult who gives a history of a sore throat which may or may not have been treated with antibiotics. After five to seven days the pain in the throat becomes worse, especially on one side. The patient is feverish and unwell, gradually he experiences more and more difficulty in opening his mouth (trismus). He may become dehydrated because

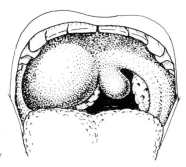

Fig. 19/3 A quinsy

of a diminished fluid intake. Swallowing becomes difficult even for saliva which may therefore dribble out of the mouth.

The mouth and throat should be examined; this is not easy because of the trismus. If there is merely inflammation and oedema around the tonsil (peritonsillitis) then a good response can be anticipated by prescribing intramuscular penicillin, 1 mega-unit, six-hourly. The patient must be encouraged to drink plenty of fluids. If he is unable to do this, intravenous fluids should be instituted.

If an abscess is found, then it must be drained. The mucous membrane on the surface of the abscess is gently painted with a local anaesthetic such as 5% cocaine solution. The abscess is then incised using the tip of a scalpel (the blade should be protected). The patient's clothing should be protected with waterproof drapes and he is given a bowl into which he can spit the pus and blood. After incision and drainage there is immediate and gratifying (to the patient) relief of symptoms.

Once the temperature has settled and the patient is better, he may be discharged to continue taking oral antibiotics at home. Arrangements should be made for the patient to undergo tonsillectomy after no more than an interval of five to six weeks. By this time the inflammation will have settled. If surgery is left for a longer time, the tonsil becomes surrounded by scar tissue and the operation becomes more difficult.

QUINSY TONSILLECTOMY

It is perfectly possible to carry out tonsillectomy as soon as a quinsy is diagnosed; however, there are hazards which may be encountered by the anaesthetist. Because of the swelling caused by the abscess it may be very difficult to see the larynx and to pass an endotracheal tube. There is also the risk of rupturing the abscess with the blade of the laryngoscope with subsequent inhalation of the pus. For these reasons delayed tonsillectomy is considered wiser by some surgeons.

Acute tonsillitis or a peritonsillar abscess may be confused with glandular fever (infectious mononucleosis). The latter may be diagnosed through a differential white blood cell count and a Paul Bunnell test.

Standard tonsillectomy

Nowadays in the United Kingdom nearly all tonsils are removed under general anaesthesia by the dissection method. The child is anaesthetised and an endotracheal tube passed. A sandbag is placed under the shoulders in order to minimise the risk of blood and secretions being aspirated into the lungs. Sterile drapes are placed around the head and across the chest. The sucker is connected and switched on. The surgeon sits at the head of the patient and wears a headlight (Fig. 19/4). A Boyle-Davis mouth gag is inserted. The tongue blade is usually split down to the middle to accommodate the endotracheal tube (Doughty tongue blade).

If the adenoids are to be removed it is usually easier to remove them first with an adenoid curette and then to insert a gauze swab into the nasopharynx until the tonsils have been removed. The gauze may then be removed and the bleeding will have stopped.

The tonsil is grasped and pulled toward the midline (Fig. 19/5). The mucous membrane along the front, top and back of the tonsil is divided with scissors. The tonsil is attached to the muscles of the pharyngeal wall by a layer of connective tissue through which blood vessels pass to the tonsil. It is a relatively easy matter to peel the tonsil away from the muscles, at the same time severing the small arteries and veins. The lower pole of the tonsil is tougher and must be divided with a wire snare.

Once one tonsil has been removed the tonsillar fossa is packed with a dry gauze swab while the other tonsil is removed.

The surgeon returns to the first tonsil: the swab is removed when it will be seen that most of the bleeding will have stopped. Any remaining bleeding points are picked up with the points of a pair of artery forceps and the vessel tied with linen or silk. Bleeding points which are particularly troublesome may have to be undersewn with a catgut suture. It is essential that at the end of the operation all bleeding has ceased.

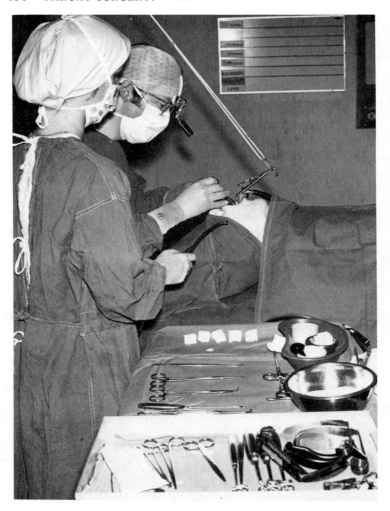

Fig. 19/4 A tonsillectomy in progress. *Note* the headlight worn by the surgeon, and the position of the instrument trolley. A Boyle-Davis gag is in position

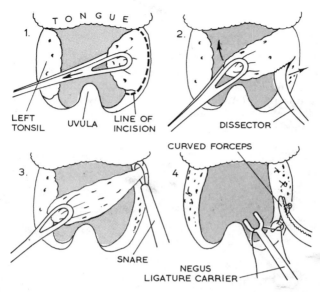

Fig. 19/5 The method of tonsillectomy surgery

Swabs and instruments are counted; all blood is sucked from the pharynx and the gag is removed. The teeth are inspected to make sure that none has been damaged by the gag.

The endotracheal tube is removed by the anaesthetist and the child is nursed on his side in the tonsil position until he has regained consciousness and is able to protect his own airway (Fig. 19/6).

SPECIFIC NURSING POINTS

Pre-operative

It is important to note whether the patient is free from any infection, and that he has not had a cold or sore throat in the two weeks prior to admission. Should infection be present there is a danger of post-operative haemorrhage.

Adequate explanation of the operation should be given to the patient or, in the case of a child, to the parents. He should be told that he will be nursed in a semi-prone position immediately post-operatively.

Postoperative

POSITIONING
Following surgery, and before the patient leaves the theatre, he is placed in a semi-prone (tonsil) position with the foot of the bed elevated (Fig. 19/6). This allows any secretions to drain freely and not be inhaled. Tonsillectomy patients usually return to the ward once they are conscious, and they will continue to be nursed in the semi-prone position but with the bed level.

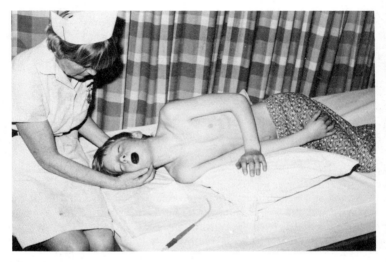

Fig. 19/6   The tonsil position

AIRWAY
The ward nurse should satisfy herself that the patient is breathing well and is rousable before letting the recovery/theatre nurse leave the ward. Gentle oral suction may be needed if the patient is still oozing blood through the mouth, but this should be done using a strict sterile procedure so as not to introduce infection to the tonsil bed.

OBSERVATIONS
On his return to the ward, the patient's pulse is taken and recorded every half hour for at least two hours. If it is stable it need not be

taken so frequently. A rise in pulse rate could indicate that the patient may be bleeding from the tonsil bed; the nurse should also keep a close watch on the patient to observe whether he is swallowing frequently. If he has swallowed a large amount of blood he may well vomit fresh blood. Medical help should be sought and the tonsil bed inspected to see which side is bleeding.

SEDATION

Following a tonsillectomy the patient should be kept as quiet and painfree as possible. Therefore sedation and analgesia are important. Some anaesthetists prefer to give an oral premedication such as atropine, and then the patient can be given an opiate immediately after surgery. Further sedation should be given as and when necessary as directed by the anaesthetist. It is important that the patient has a good night's sleep postoperatively as the throat is very sore. Once the patient is able to take fluids by mouth, soluble aspirin gargles, which can be swallowed, should be given. If he is unable to take aspirin, soluble paracetamol is just as effective. The oral analgesics should be given half an hour before meals to ease the sore throat.

DIET AND FLUIDS

It is usual to give nothing by mouth for four to six hours postoperatively; cubes of ice to suck are soothing. Once fluids can be tolerated, eating may be commenced. It is important to encourage chewing and swallowing early so the back of the throat does not become stiff and swollen. Cornflakes, crisps and apples are all good examples of crisp food which should be eaten. Fluids should be taken in abundance.

ORAL TOILET

After about six hours, cold mouthwashes can be given and the front teeth gently cleaned. Once diet is begun, saline or hydrogen peroxide gargles should be given after food to help to clean the tonsil bed from any food which may adhere to it.

CONVALESCENT CARE AND DISCHARGE FROM HOSPITAL

The patient usually remains in hospital for three to five days postoperatively. Once the tonsil bed looks clean and healthy and the patient is eating and drinking well he may go home. He should be advised to remain away from work/school for about 14 days from the day of operation. It is advisable to continue with aspirin gargles before meals and salt gargles afterwards. Sometimes patients experience earache and they should be advised to put cotton wool in their ears when washing their hair. For at least two weeks after the operation they should not go swimming or enter crowded places such as shops, pubs, discos, etc., where they might catch a cold.

Nursing problems

Following tonsillectomy the nurse should be alert to the possibility of any of the following:

HAEMORRHAGE

This can be either *reactionary* or *secondary*. Reactionary haemorrhage starts within hours of the operation, while secondary haemorrhage usually occurs five to seven days postoperatively.

Reactionary haemorrhage: A patient may commence bleeding after having returned to the ward. A pad soaked in adrenaline, then wrung out, should be applied firmly to the bleeding point by the doctor; this may be sufficient to control the haemorrhage. If it fails, or the patient is a child, he will then have to go back to theatre to have the bleeding point ligated. Preparations must be made for an intravenous drip to be set up, and blood should be taken for cross-matching.

On return to the ward the patient will have a blood transfusion in progress, or a saline infusion.

An important note here concerns the admission assessment. All patients who are admitted for tonsillectomy should be asked what is their religion. Jehovah's Witnesses do not allow blood transfusions and the doctor should be aware whether the patient is a Jehovah's Witness, in the event of bleeding.

Secondary haemorrhage: If a patient begins to bleed five to seven days following tonsillectomy he must be readmitted to hospital. The cause of the bleeding is almost always an infection in the tonsil bed. An intravenous infusion is commenced and antibiotics given intravenously for 24–48 hours. A blood transfusion may be required.

The patient remains in bed until the bleeding stops. Hydrogen peroxide gargles should be given (5–10ml of H_2O_2 in a mug of water) as they will help to disperse any old clot, or slough, from the tonsil bed. Once the tonsil bed looks healthy and no further bleeding has occurred for at least 48 hours, the patient may return home and continue with oral antibiotics.

PYREXIA

Sometimes patients will develop a temperature postoperatively. If this persists over 24 hours, it is advisable that they commence anti-biotics to prevent infection developing in the tonsil bed with the possibility of secondary haemorrhage occurring.

RELUCTANCE WITH DIET AND FLUIDS

Some patients are very reluctant to eat and drink because the throat is so sore; this becomes a vicious circle as the less they swallow the more sore the throat becomes. The nurse must have patience, yet be firm with such patients, encouraging them to eat and drink, little and often.

EARACHE

Following a tonsillectomy the patient often suffers acute earache. Aspirin or paracetamol given for the throat soreness should help to relieve the earache as well.

ADENOIDECTOMY (Fig. 19/7)

The adenoid is a collection of lymphoid tissue situated on the pos-terior wall of the nasopharynx and lying close to the openings of the

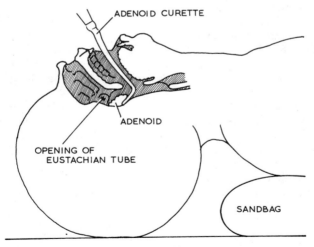

Fig. 19/7 Adenoidectomy, showing the curette

Eustachian tubes. The adenoid is present at birth and usually enlarges between the ages of three and five after which it first stops enlarging and then gradually shrinks. As the child continues growing the size of the adenoid relative to the size of the nasopharynx becomes less and less.

If the adenoid becomes large it may block the posterior opening of the nose causing nasal obstruction, mouth breathing and snoring at night. Nasal secretions are held up and may become infected. This infection may spread up the Eustachian tube and give rise to otitis media (see p. 52).

Obstruction of the Eustachian tube by an enlarged adenoid is a common accompaniment of secretory otitis media. Adenoids which are relatively large and which are giving rise to symptoms should be surgically removed under general anaesthesia.

The child is placed in the tonsil position and the mouth is held open with a Boyle-Davis gag (see Fig. 19/4). The adenoid is removed from behind the soft palate using a curette. A gauze swab is placed behind the soft palate to control the bleeding which usually stops after two or three minutes. The gauze is then removed.

The operation of adenoidectomy is often combined with tonsillectomy or with myringotomies and insertion of grommets.

Specific nursing points

The general plan of nursing care is as for tonsillectomy, with one most important addition.

If the child has a severe haemorrhage in theatre or a reactionary haemorrhage in the ward which results in his being taken back to theatre, it may be necessary to insert a *post-nasal pack* to stop the bleeding (Fig. 19/8).

This pack takes the form of a gauze roll to which three tapes are securely fastened. One tape comes out through each nostril and the two tapes are tied over the columella preventing the pack from slipping down into the throat. The third tape comes out through the mouth and may be taped to the cheek.

When the child returns from theatre an intravenous infusion will be in progress. The child will need to be sedated as the pack is not very comfortable.

REMOVAL OF POST-NASAL PACK

This is quite a simple procedure which is carried out on the ward

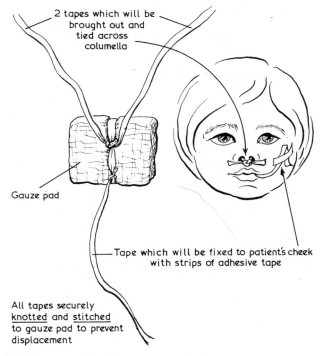

2 tapes which will be
brought out and
tied across
columella

Gauze pad

Tape which will be fixed to patient's cheek
with strips of adhesive tape

All tapes securely
knotted and stitched
to gauze pad to prevent
displacement

Fig. 19/8 A post-nasal pack

by the doctor. All that are required:
A pair of sharp scissors
Kidney dish
Some gauze or tissues
The nurse supports the child's head gently but firmly. The doctor carefully cuts the two tapes holding the pack in place, and cuts off the knot. The child opens his mouth and the surgeon slips his finger into the mouth along the third tape attached to the pack. Using gentle downward traction on the tape the pack is delivered through the mouth. The infusion will remain in position until later the same day in case any further bleeding occurs.

Laryngeal Carcinoma: Laryngectomy

Cancer of the larynx is the most common cancer seen in ENT surgery. The majority of carcinomas arise on the vocal cords (Fig. 20/1) giving rise to the most important symptom – hoarseness. As the tumour grows larger it may narrow the airway, leading to difficulties with breathing or stridor (noisy breathing). The condition is not usually painful until the tumour is well advanced when it may also bleed. The patient may cough up blood, haemoptysis.

Any person who suffers hoarseness which lasts for more than three to four weeks without showing signs of improvement should be referred to an ENT surgeon so that his larynx can be examined. In the clinic, it is usually possible to examine the larynx with a mirror (indirect laryngoscopy), (see Fig. 1/2, p. 3). If the larynx cannot

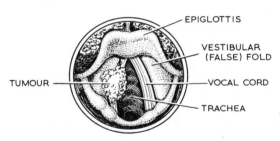

Fig. 20/1 Tumour of the larynx showing the growth on a vocal cord

be seen properly, or if something abnormal has been seen, then the patient should be admitted for a direct laryngoscopy under general anaesthetic. At the same time a biopsy can be taken for examination.

If the biopsy confirms a malignant tumour a decision has to be taken as to the best form of treatment. This is best done by a combined consultation between the ENT surgeon, a radiotherapist and the patient with his family.

The choice of treatment must be tailored to the requirements of the individual patient, and requires consideration of many factors including the patient's age and state of health, the site and size of the tumour, and the nature of any proposed surgery to remove the tumour.

In general terms, small tumours will do well with radiotherapy whereas larger tumours, or tumours which have spread to involve the lymph nodes of the neck, tend to do better with surgery. If radiotherapy fails to cure the tumour, then laryngectomy (removal of the larynx) will be considered.

LARYNGECTOMY (Fig. 20/2)

Removal of the larynx means the end of normal talking. It is not lightly undertaken and the patient must be well prepared beforehand. The surgeon will need to explain carefully the implications of the operation. If possible a visit from someone who has undergone surgery and has learned to speak again may be helpful.

The speech therapist should be introduced at the very earliest time. It is useful for her to hear how the patient speaks; has he an accent or an impediment; is he fluent in speaking, etc. It is also important to know whether the patient can read or write. A few years ago inability to read or write would have meant that the patient would be totally unable to communicate postoperatively. Under these circumstances the wisdom of surgery should be seriously considered. Nowadays communication at an early stage is possible post-surgery with the help of specialised mechanical vibrators provided by the speech therapist.

After the larynx has been removed the end of the trachea is brought out on to the front of the neck, to provide a permanent opening (tracheostome) for breathing. The remaining part of the food channel, the pharynx, is stitched together to make a tube so that the patient will be able to swallow normally. A nasogastric tube is then passed down through a nostril into the pharynx and on to the stomach. This allows the patient to be fed while the pharynx heals. This normally takes about 10 days.

The skin incision is sutured and drains inserted. If the wound is not drained blood may accumulate forming a haematoma which may become infected. Antibiotics are usually prescribed.

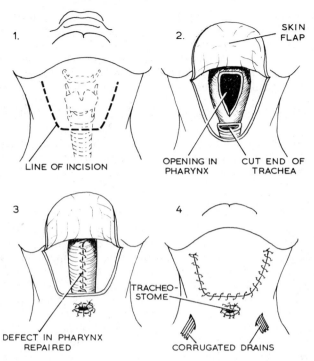

1.

LINE OF INCISION

2.

SKIN
FLAP

OPENING IN
PHARYNX

CUT END OF
TRACHEA

3

DEFECT IN PHARYNX
REPAIRED

4

TRACHEO-
STOME

CORRUGATED DRAINS

Fig. 20/2 Laryngectomy

A tracheostomy tube with an inflatable cuff is inserted into the tracheostome. The cuff is usually inflated for the first 12 hours to prevent blood from dribbling down the trachea into the lungs.

Humidification must be provided to prevent the formation of crusts of dried mucus. If large crusts are allowed to form they may eventually block the trachea.

Excess secretions are removed by gentle suction. Breathing exercises are given by the physiotherapist.

The drains are removed from the neck when drainage stops, usually after about two days. The tracheostomy tube is changed as often as necessary, usually daily.

The stitches are removed from the skin incision and from around the stoma when the wounds are well healed, between the 7th and 10th postoperative days.

Table 20/1 **Immediate postoperative care plan following laryngectomy**

Problem	Goal/objective	Care/action	Evaluation
1. Possible airway obstruction	Maintain clear airway	$\frac{1}{2}$- to 1-hourly suction Continuous humidification	Breathing comfortable No sign(s) of distress
2. Possible shock, either from the anaesthetic or through haemorrhage	Observations Stable condition, no bleeding	$\frac{1}{2}$-hourly blood pressure and pulse Check neck and stoma and drainage bottles for excess bleeding	Observations stable – may be done less frequently No visible signs of bleeding or shock
3. Pain	To keep the patient pain-free	Regular postoperative analgesia Watch position of the patient's head and neck	No complaints Keep analgesics regular
4. Unable to have oral fluids	Maintain fluid intake	Intravenous infusion in progress Strict fluid balance chart	Satisfactory fluid intake
5. Dry mouth	Keep mouth moist and fresh	Regular mouth care four-hourly	Mouth comfortable at present
6. Communication anxiety	Establish good communication	Provide patient with pen and paper/Magic writer Continual reassurance	Patient able to make himself understood Shows no sign(s) of anxiety
7. Possible urine retention	Pass urine normally	Watch output carefully and chart Offer bottle/bedpan ? requires catheterisation	Has passed urine – no need to catheterise
8. Mobility	Prevent DVT To achieve full mobility as soon as possible	Bed rest at present Encourage leg movements two-hourly Change of position two-hourly	Good mobility in bed No sign(s) of DVT or pressure sores

When all the stitches are out the nasogastric feeding tube may be removed and the patient given first, liquids and then soft solids to eat by mouth. At this stage the speech therapist may start to teach the patient oesophageal speech.

Table 20/1 gives an example of an immediate postoperative care plan.

CHAPTER TWENTY-ONE

Block Dissection of the Cervical Lymph Nodes

The lymphatic supply of the head and neck is rich, and drains ultimately to the cervical lymph nodes (see Fig. 16/11, p. 135). Most head and neck tumours will metastasise at some stage to the cervical lymph nodes. Tumours which arise from structures with a poor lymphatic drainage, such as the vocal cords, will metastasise late; structures which have a rich lymphatic supply, such as the tongue, will metastasise early.

Lymph nodes which become enlarged and hard due to the presence of malignant tumour may be treated by radiotherapy, chemotherapy, surgery, or by a combination of these. A block dissection (i.e. the removal of the deep and superficial chains of nodes) may have to be carried out in conjunction with removal of the primary tumour, e.g. a laryngeal cancer which has metastasised.

OPERATIVE PROCEDURE (Figs. 21/1, 21/2)

A general anaesthetic is administered and maintained either with an endotracheal tube or through a tracheostomy if there has been any airway obstruction, for instance by a large tumour.

The operation involves removal of the cervical chain of lymph nodes together with the internal jugular vein and the overlying sternomastoid muscle. After the skin incisions have been made the skin flaps are raised. All the superficial tissues of the neck are removed down to the level of the fascia covering the deep muscles of the neck. The neck is cleared from the midline anteriorly to the trapezius muscle posteriorly and from the level of the clavicle up to the level of the mandible. The submandibular salivary gland should also be removed although it may be permissible to leave the gland if the involved lymph nodes arise lower in the neck away from the submandibular region. The carotid artery and vagus nerve are left.

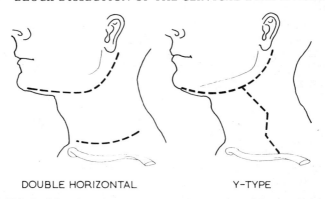

DOUBLE HORIZONTAL   Y-TYPE

Fig. 21/1 Incision for carrying out a block dissection of the cervical lymph nodes

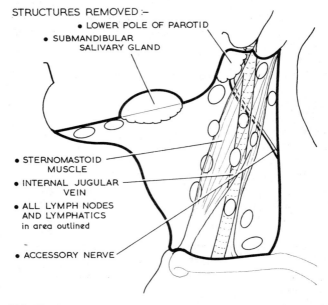

Fig. 21/2 To show the structures removed in a block dissection of cervical lymph nodes. *Note* the relationship of the accessory nerve

At the end of the operation haemostasis is carefully secured. The skin edges are sutured and drains are inserted to prevent the formation of a haematoma beneath the skin flaps. Any fluid which collects beneath the wound should be aspirated using an aseptic technique. It is important that the skin flaps adhere securely to the underlying tissues from which they can then derive an additional blood supply.

Complications
1. If the neck skin becomes infected or undergoes necrosis, there is a real risk that the underlying unprotected carotid artery will rupture with a fatal outcome. This is more likely to occur following radiotherapy.
2. The trapezius muscle is mainly supplied by the accessory nerve (XIth cranial) which passes through the sternomastoid muscle. As the sternomastoid is removed the nerve is cut. This means that the patient's shoulder will tend to droop unless active shoulder shrugging exercises are encouraged. The physiotherapist will have taught the exercises pre-operatively. The trapezius muscle does have a supplementary muscle supply which will, to some extent, take over the role of the accessory nerve. It is for this reason that exercises should be encouraged as soon as possible.

NURSING NOTES

Pre-operative
Explanation The nurse must ensure that the doctor has explained fully to the patient the nature of the operation. It is helpful if she can ascertain that the patient has fully understood. If the patient has any doubts or fears he is more likely to confide in the nurse. The nurse should endeavour to answer any questions, but if she is not able she must ask the doctor to return and discuss the matter further with the patient.
Shave Any hair in the direct operative field should be shaved. This will involve an area from the mastoid process to the chest and, in the case of a male, extending to the nipple line. If a split-skin graft is to be used, the donor area on the thigh should be shaved also.

Postoperative
Airway At all times the nurse must ensure that the patient's airway is unobstructed and free from secretions or bleeding. If the block

dissection is done at the same time as the removal of the primary tumour, the patient may have a temporary or permanent tracheostomy (depending on the site of the tumour). Care of the tracheostomy is described in Chapter 18.

Position The sternomastoid muscle supports the head and neck. It is removed during the operation and consequently the patient's head and neck will need to be well supported by correctly placed pillows.

Observations The nurse should make regular observations of the pulse, blood pressure, respiration rate and the temperature.

Wound care Large skin flaps are raised in order that the operative field is adequately exposed. After the operation it is important to prevent the formation of a haematoma beneath the flaps so that the wounds will heal satisfactorily. If a haematoma is allowed to collect the blood supply to the flaps may be cut off and the skin would die. The nurse must look carefully at any drains which may be in the wound to ensure that they drain adequately and do not become dislodged. If they cease to work the doctor must be notified.

Pain control Adequate analgesia should be given to control any pain or discomfort.

Fluids Intravenous fluids will have been commenced in the operating theatre and these should be continued until the patient can tolerate nasogastric fluids or, if permitted, oral fluids. A fluid balance chart must be kept.

Care after the first 24 hours

The patient's head and neck will need to be carefully supported. Regular charting of the temperature, pulse and respiration rate should continue.

Suction drains will remain in situ until there is less than 10ml drainage in 24 hours. They are removed using an aseptic technique. Nasogastric feeds or a light nourishing diet will be given as appropriate. Analgesia should be given according to the individual patient's needs.

Physiotherapy will be given regularly, both breathing and vibrations to encourage expectoration of any secretions, and gentle shoulder shrugging exercises to avoid stiffening of the shoulder girdle. Head and neck posture will probably need retraining to avoid the head's being held on one side because of the removal of the sternomastoid muscle – a mirror is helpful. As the patient becomes more active so exercises may be increased. Shoulder shrugging exercises should be continued for several months after the patient goes home – the accessory nerve which supplies the trapezius muscle will almost certainly have been divided and the supplementary nerve supply will need to be encouraged to take over.

Nursing problems

HAEMORRHAGE

If there is bleeding beneath the skin flaps the first sign may be swelling of the wound site. Alternatively fresh blood may be seen leaking through the wound or through the drains. The doctor must be notified. Slight oozing may be controlled by a firm pressure dressing; for more substantial bleeding the patient may have to return to the theatre for ligation of the bleeding point.

If the patient has previously had irradiation to the neck; any infection in the tissues of the neck; any leakage of saliva containing digestive enzymes into the neck; or if there is residual tumour in the neck, the carotid artery, or one of its branches, is at risk. In such cases very brisk arterial bleeding demands urgent attention: firm digital pressure should be applied over the bleeding point and maintained until assistance arrives, when the patient should be taken immediately to the operating theatre and the artery clamped.

HEALING

If the patient has undergone radiotherapy or chemotherapy, healing of the wound may be delayed. The neck wound may break down and require skin grafting which will delay the patient's discharge.

DEEP VEIN THROMBOSIS

Although most patients can be encouraged to be up and about after 24 hours, there will be some who are not able to be so active. These include the patient with severe arthritis. In such patients there is a greater risk of developing a deep vein thrombosis (DVT) and he should be fitted with anti-embolism stockings.

SUTURES

Alternate sutures are usually removed after seven days and the remainder the following day. In cases where there has been irradiation involving the wound site, sutures may be left for a longer period.

CHAPTER TWENTY-TWO

Removal of Foreign Bodies

Most ENT operations are non-urgent but there are some emergency procedures. Tracheostomy is one such procedure (see Chapter 18). The other common emergency concerns the swallowing/inhalation/ insertion of foreign bodies via various orifices. Sharp or bulky objects may become accidentally lodged in the pharynx or oesophagus of an adult; children or mentally subnormal adults may poke small objects into the nose or ear canal.

NOSE

Any foreign body retained in the nose for more than a few hours, especially if it consists of vegetable material, will act as an irritant

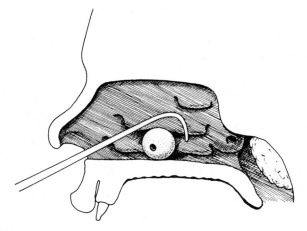

Fig. 22/1 Removal of a foreign body from the nose

and give rise to a unilateral nasal discharge which quickly becomes infected.

If the child is co-operative and the object is easily visible, the foreign body may be removed in the doctor's surgery or in the casualty department. Otherwise the child should be admitted to hospital and the offending object removed under a general anaesthetic. Soft objects such as pieces of tissue paper or sponge rubber may be grasped with nasal forceps, but hard or smooth objects such as beads or buttons must be dealt with differently. If an attempt is made to grasp the object with forceps then the object is bound to slip and be pushed even farther back. A hooked instrument is passed beyond the object and then gently pulled forward, bringing the foreign body with it (Fig. 22/1).

EAR

An unskilled person should not attempt to remove a foreign body from the ear of a struggling child because there is a real danger of damaging the tympanic membrane and ossicles. The child should be admitted; under general anaesthesia the object should be removed in the same way as from the nose. The operating microscope may be used.

The ear canal and tympanic membrane should be carefully inspected afterwards for any signs of damage to these delicate structures. An ear dressing of 1.25cm ($\frac{1}{2}$in) ribbon gauze soaked in a steroid-containing ear preparation such as Otosporin may be inserted, and removed after 24 hours. Some objects, such as insects, which occasionally crawl into the ear canal, may be removed by syringing.

When removing a foreign body from the nose or ear of a child, the surgeon should always look in the other nostril or ear canal for unsuspected objects.

SWALLOWED FOREIGN BODIES

Sharp objects, such as pieces of bone, are occasionally accidentally taken into the mouth with food and swallowed. This tends to happen more in people who wear false teeth and who therefore, may not feel the object in the mouth until it is too late.

The most common site for such objects to become lodged is at the level of the crico-pharyngeal sphincter. The condition may be so painful that the patient cannot even swallow his own saliva. Examination by indirect laryngoscopy may show the upper end of the foreign body sticking up behind the larynx, but more commonly the only thing to be seen is pooling of saliva in the pharynx. The neck may be tender to palpation.

A lateral radiograph of the neck may show the foreign body (if it is radio-opaque) but many fish bones and pieces of cartilage do not show up. A clear history that a foreign body has been swallowed and become lodged is more important than a negative radiograph. If there is any doubt at all, the patient should be examined under a general anaesthetic. The risk of leaving a foreign body is that it may pierce the thin wall of the pharynx and give rise to a parapharyngeal abscess. This in turn may spread downward into the chest and give rise to a fatal mediastinitis.

The pharynx and oesophagus are carefully inspected under direct vision (oesophagoscopy). As soon as the foreign body is located it is grasped with suitably long forceps and gently withdrawn, taking special care not to damage further the mucosal lining of the pharynx or oesophagus.

The patient's recovery from anaesthesia must be closely supervised. The nurse should watch for any signs of shock, such as pallor, cold clammy skin, a rising pulse or a falling blood pressure; for a rise in temperature; or signs of air in the tissues of the neck. This is known as surgical emphysema and feels like eggshell crackling beneath the skin. If any of these signs is present, or if the patient complains of pain in the back or chest, this may indicate that the pharynx or oesophagus has been perforated. This demands urgent surgical exploration and repair of the perforation.

Following removal of a foreign body from the throat, it is safer to starve the patient for at least six hours, or overnight, and then to give only sterile water by mouth, provided that none of the features described above contra-indicate this. If the sterile water is tolerated well, the patient may be given more substantial food until he is taking a full diet once more.

CHAPTER TWENTY-THREE

The Role of Other Professionals

Ear, nose and throat surgeons do not work in isolation. Apart from the nursing staff and medical colleagues there are other professionals involved in the overall care and rehabilitation of patients. These include the physiotherapist and occupational therapist; the diagnostic and therapeutic radiographer; and in some cases the dental prosthetist. Particularly involved can be the speech therapist, hearing therapist and social worker and it is the work of these three that will be described in this chapter.

SPEECH THERAPY

Speech therapy is particularly necessary after laryngectomy; in cases where there is evidence of vocal strain; and, more rarely, in instances of non-organic voice disorders.

Laryngectomy

The speech therapist is one of the team who is concerned with the total rehabilitation of the patient who undergoes laryngectomy, and this includes the development of communication using a substitute voice. Ideally the speech therapist will see the patient pre-operatively and explain to him about oesophageal voice; the technique to achieve this is discussed and sometimes the patient may wish to meet someone who is a confident pseudo-voice speaker. At this early stage the speech therapist will be able to assess how much the patient has understood the implications of the operation and the stages of recovery. Any misunderstandings should be reported to the medical or nursing staff, and cleared up before the operation.

Immediately after surgery regular visits by the speech therapist are important in preparing the patient for actual voice work. He or she should be encouraged to communicate by *gentle* mouthing: *forced* whispering may lead to tension developing and this is to be avoided as it may impair subsequent attempts at voice production.

As soon as the tissues of the pharynx are healed, with no evidence of a fistula, the nasogastric tube is removed and oesophageal voice can be attempted. The patient is taught to take air through the mouth and squeeze it back into the oesophagus bringing it forward again to vibrate in the throat making a characteristic belching sound. Some patients find this easy and soon develop a controlled voice. Unfortunately, many never acquire voice, but these patients should not be considered failures. There are a number of electronic voice vibrators available which, after careful training, will allow adequate communication. For some patients learning to use one of these is an achievement in itself. Success or failure should really be judged by a person's own adjustment to a new kind of voice whether it be oesophageal or electronic.

The speech therapist's involvement with a laryngectomy patient may continue for many months.

Vocal strain

Vocal strain occurs because of the way an individual produces his or her voice. Ultimately it can result in organic changes in the larynx such as vocal cord oedema or nodules, and does require vocal re-education. Different working conditions and lifestyles make different demands upon the vocal apparatus; some people make the necessary adjustments for these demands but others need help.

Anxiety and stress are frequently reflected in inadequate voice production. Recognition of these causes together with practical exercises in correct voice production will often prevent organic changes. If changes have already necessitated surgery, voice therapy can prevent such changes recurring. Most of these patients require only short-term treatment.

Non-organic voice disorder

The speech therapist's role is limited in the treatment of the more deep-seated psychological disturbance, where there may be the symptoms of voice disorder. Referral to other disciplines, for example psychiatrist or psychologist may be necessary.

HEARING THERAPY

Hearing therapists are the newest professional group within audiology services, if not the National Health Service as a whole. They were introduced in 1979 as part of a programme to improve rehabilitation services for deafened adults. Generally, audiology services in this country have been technical rather than rehabilitative, with medical and surgical expertise widely available, as well as an extensive system for the supply and fitting of hearing aids. Until recent years there has been far less concern or provision for the very considerable number of people who cannot be helped by surgical intervention, or whose problems are not ameliorated by the unsupported issue of a hearing aid.

The use of a hearing aid is not a simple matter of compensating hearing loss by amplification. The supply of a hearing aid should be the beginning of a service. In addition to correct fitting, suitable advice and training must be available. Not only the ears, but the personality, lifestyle, age and attitude of the aid–user is involved.

The therapist's aim is to help the hearing-impaired person come to terms with his handicap, and then to develop skills to alleviate the adverse results of hearing loss so that he can continue to function within his social and occupational competency. If the person is to function adequately an understanding of the implications of hearing loss and the ways in which hearing aids, lip-reading and auditory training can help are vital. A programme designed to maximise a patient's ability to communicate will be formulated by the therapist. This programme will seek to provide guidance and help regarding use of hearing aids and environmental aids; lip-reading instruction and auditory training; tactics for coping in noisy listening situations; advice to the family; and, when appropriate in the case of the elderly and physically handicapped, domiciliary visits.

Only a small number of hearing therapists work within the NHS, and at present it is not possible for every adult with acquired hearing loss to be referred to one.

THE ROLE OF THE SOCIAL WORKER IN THE ENT DEPARTMENT

Types of work

The social worker in the ENT department will find that some patients present problems common to all social work, for example low self-esteem may cause difficulties in adjusting to new demands; poor family relationships can result in an inability to accept help.

Some patients lack a knowledge of services available or the skills to obtain them.

Patients may present symptoms of the stress caused by disease or the experience of hospital admission. Behaviour can vary from an inability to mention difficulties or ask appropriate and worrying questions, to an unwillingness to participate in therapy or to a misunderstanding of procedures. The extent of the stress is sometimes missed by the medical/nursing staff, and the social worker may become aware of this as it is essential for her to understand the patients's normal standing in his community.

There are also the problems inherent in the disease or of the treatment itself. For instance, the relatives may have a deep fear of radiotherapy, or of learning new skills associated with the care of a tracheostomy. If the larynx is involved the patient and relatives may need to consider the particular loneliness and frustrations which may arise. Chronic ear infections may be associated with a drop in self-confidence leading to employment problems and family disharmony.

Less frequently there are problems associated with disfigurement especially of the face and the neck. Patients need to be able to express their ambivalence towards the scar, perhaps encouragement to socialise and to be reassured by recognition of their own uniqueness and social value.

Using the social worker
When considering which patients might be referred to the social worker it may be easier to think of vulnerable groups. Obviously even within these groups not everyone needs referring but might well benefit from careful consideration by ward staff. At all times the social worker attempts to help the individual make the best use of his own abilities and respects his right to make his own choices and decisions. It is expected that he is told of the proposed referral. Patients who may be referred include:

The frail elderly patient living alone or with an equally frail elderly spouse. Even concerned loving families may be too scattered to offer adequate practical support. Domiciliary services, residential or day care may be necesssry on discharge.

Patients having surgery resulting in disfigurement or speech impairment. All laryngectomy patients should be seen by the social worker before surgery and prior to discharge, thus providing him an opportunity to express anxiety about the future and to receive the reassurance of an easily available and understanding source of assistance.

The interview prior to surgery is often used by the patient to reassure himself of his individual worth by a review of his life's successes. When discussing discharge plans it is useful to consider reactions of family and friends and methods of dealing with frustrations.

What the social worker offers
1. *Mobilisation of practical help:*
   Home help or other domiciliary services
   Financial assistance via grants or benefits
   Advice re accommodation problems
   Community service, e.g. day care, social activities
   Residential care
2. Emotional support and the opportunity to consider difficulties and any necessary adjustments or plans; by encouraging discussion and by offering careful listening.
3. *Knowledge of other facilities and how to obtain them:*
   Voluntary organisations
   National insurance benefits
   Private residential care
   Local authority services
4. Understanding of the social and psychological processes involved in coping with stress which may be of assistance in making assessments or treatment plans.

Social worker as a member of the ENT team
In order to use the professional skills of the social worker it is helpful to be familiar with her method of work, especially how she makes an assessment. Personal contact between medical and nursing staff and the social worker is especially valuable.

The social worker will also make demands on the team:
1. She needs information about the disease and treatment plan, and to be kept up to date and given warning of discharge dates.
2. She needs time. While the importance of an early referral cannot be over-emphasised it is often not until the patient nears the end of his course of treatment that his domestic or social needs can be assessed. Consequent plans may require time to bring them to fruition, and the social worker may ask for the discharge date to reflect this.

3. She needs privacy. The patient will be encouraged to examine his feelings which may be ambivalent or painful. He may need to discuss his financial situation, his fears and some confidential matters. This cannot be done in an open ward even with the privacy of curtains. Normally, the social worker will ask to see the patient in a separate room without interruptions.

CHAPTER TWENTY-FOUR

Drugs and Other Substances used in ENT

ANALGESICS

These are preparations used for the relief of pain.

Mild to moderate pain

Aspirin is the drug of choice for headache and is widely used following tonsillectomy. It also has anti–inflammatory properties which may be useful. Gastric irritation may be a problem. It is cheap.

Paracetamol is as effective but has no demonstrable anti–inflammatory activity. Paediatric paracetamol elixir is preferable to aspirin in infants. Both aspirin and paracetamol are antipyrexial.

Moderate to severe pain

Codeine, *dihydrocodeine* and *pentazocine* may all be used, but for additional information including the side–effects and hazards the reader should refer to the *British National Formulary*.

Narcotics and other analgesics used for severe pain

With repeated administration they cause tolerance and dependence and all cause constipation by decreasing intestinal mobility.

Morphine remains a valuable narcotic analgesic for severe pain but may cause nausea and vomiting. It often confers a state of euphoria and mental detachment which may enhance the sense of well-being.

Diamorphine (heroin) is more likely to produce euphoria and addiction but is less likely to make the patient feel sick.

Methadone is less sedating than morphine and is useful for providing background pain relief in terminal disease.

Drugs used for the relief of postoperative pain
Papaveretum is a mixture of opium alkaloids containing morphine and may be given by injection in the postoperative period. *Pethidine* may be similarly used.

ANTIBIOTICS

Precise identification of the organism causing an infection and the appropriate antibiotic to prescribe can be discovered by laboratory examination of infected material, e.g. throat or ear swab. However, in many infections one antibiotic can usually be chosen as the most likely to be effective (see below).

Infection	First choice antibiotic	Alternative
Otitis media	amoxycillin	erythromycin co-trimoxazole
Tonsillitis	penicillin	erythromycin
Sinusitis	amoxycillin	erythromycin metronidazole if anaerobic bacteria present

ANTIHISTAMINES

Antihistamines taken by mouth are of potential value in the treatment of nasal allergies, particularly the seasonal type (hay fever). There are many antihistamines available and they differ in their duration of action and the incidence of side-effects, such as drowsiness. Patients vary widely in their response to them. More recently-introduced preparations claim to cause less drowsiness.

BIPP

Bismuth and iodoform paraffin paste. It is mildly antiseptic. Ribbon gauze impregnated with BIPP is used for nasal packing to control bleeding.

EAR DROPS

For softening wax:
Sodium bicarbonate, olive oil or almond oil are very effective and
unlikely to cause irritation. Many proprietary preparations contain
organic solvents which may cause irritation of the meatal skin.

For otitis externa:
These can only be effective if the ear canal has been thoroughly
cleaned by suction, dry mopping or gentle syringing. The applica-
tion, on 1.25cm ($\frac{1}{2}$in) ribbon gauze, of an astringent such as *alumi-
nium acetate* or an *anti-inflammatory corticosteroid* solution is effective. If infection is present a topical anti-infective agent may be used,
usually in combination with a steroid. The latter reduces inflammation and also lessens itching. Combinations in common use are:
clioquinol and steroid (Locorten-Vioform); gentamicin and hydro-
cortisone (Gentisone HC); and neomycin, polymyxin, and hydrocor-
tisone (Otosporin).

The prolonged use of antibiotic ear drops should be avoided if
possible because of the risk of development of a fungal infection.

INHALATIONS

The inhalation of steam is comforting in acute infections of the nose
and throat and following nasal surgery. Inhalations will help to loosen
secretions and soften crusts. The addition of volatile substances such
as menthol and eucalyptus makes the inhalations more pleasant.

LOCAL ANAESTHETICS

Lignocaine and cocaine are effectively absorbed from the mucous
membrane and so are useful surface anaesthetics in the nose or
throat. The action of lignocaine may be prolonged by adding adrenalin, a vasoconstrictor which diminishes local blood flow and so slows
the rate of absorption. Lignocaine is available as a 2–4% solution
and is also available in gel form for anaesthetising the mouth or
throat.

Cocaine is a vasoconstrictor as well as a local anaesthetic so does
not need to be mixed with adrenalin. Maximum dose of cocaine is
3mg/kg and if the dose is exceeded there is the risk of central nervous
stimulation resulting in convulsion. Cocaine is available as a 5–10%
solution or 25% paste.

MOUTHWASHES

Mouthwashes have a mechanical cleansing action and freshen the mouth. *Thymol glycerine compound*, *hydrogen peroxide* and *sodium chloride* are equally effective.

NASAL DROPS – EPHEDRINE 0.5% OR 1%

Nasal drops act by constriction of the nasal mucosal blood vessels thereby reducing the thickness of the nasal mucosa. They are of limited value as they give rise to a secondary vasodilatation as the effect of the drug wears off. This happens after prolonged use, i.e. more than about 10 days. They provide useful symptomatic relief from nasal congestion following intranasal or sinus surgery.

NASAL SPRAYS

Many proprietary sprays contain a vasoconstrictor which prevents their long-term use (see ephedrine nasal drops). Patients with severe symptoms of nasal allergy can now expect relief from topical preparations of corticosteroid, e.g. beclomethasone, or sodium cromoglycate. Benefit from treatment depends on regular use and in some cases treatment may be continued for months or even years.

NASEPTIN CREAM

Cream containing chlorhexidine hydrochloride 0.1% and neomycin sulphate 0.5% is an anti-infective agent for the treatment of staphylococcal infection of the nasal vestibular skin. It may be used in the treatment of vestibulitis or following cauterisation of the nose for epistaxis where it will soften any crusts in the nose and allow crusts to separate without trauma or bleeding.

SILVER NITRATE

This is a caustic chemical. A 10% solution applied on cotton wool is used to cauterise granulation tissue, for example on the skin or in a mastoid cavity. Solid silver nitrate may be used to cauterise nasal blood vessels in treatment of epistaxis. *Be careful:* If silver nitrate touches the skin it burns the skin and leaves a black mark which eventually wears off.

Further Reading

ABC of Ear, Nose and Throat (1981). British Medical Association, London.

British National Formulary. Published six-monthly by the British Medical Association and the Pharmaceutical Society of Great Britain (jointly).

Bull, T.R. (1980). *Colour Atlas of ENT Diagnosis*. Wolfe Medical and Scientific Publications, London.

Bull, T.R. and Cook, J.L. (1976). *Speech Therapy and ENT Surgery*. Blackwell Scientific Publications Limited, Oxford.

Foxen, E.H.M. (1981). *Lecture Notes on Diseases of the Ear, Nose and Throat*, 5th edition. Blackwell Scientific Publications Limited, Oxford.

Hopkins, S.J. (1985). *Principal Drugs*, 8th edition. Faber and Faber, London.

Long, R. (1981). *Systematic Nursing Care*. Faber and Faber, London.

Maran, A.G.D. and Stell, P.M. (1979). *Clinical Otolaryngology*. Blackwell Scientific Publications Limited, Oxford.

Marshall, S. and Oxlade, Z.E. (jt eds) (1972). *Ear, Nose and Throat Nursing*, 5th edition. Ballière Tindall, Eastbourne.

Pracy, R., Seigler, J., Stell, P.M. and Rogers, J. (1977). *Ear, Nose and Throat Surgery and Nursing*. Hodder and Stoughton, Sevenoaks.

Serra, A.M., Bailey, C.M. and Jackson, P.D. (1982). *Ear, Nose and Throat Nursing*. Blackwell Scientific Publications Limited, Oxford.

Shaw, P. (1985). *The Deaf CAN Speak*. Faber and Faber, London.

Has Voice - Will Speak by Vera Tait LCST is a useful book for anyone wishing to learn more about oesophageal speech, or recommend to someone who has undergone laryngectomy. It may be purchased from the author at Old Coastguards, West Appledore, Bideford, Devon EX39 1SB.

Useful Organisations

The Royal National Institute for the Deaf
105 Gower Street
London WC1E 6AH   01-387 8033

The National Deaf Children's Society
45 Hereford Road
London W2 5AH   01-229 9272

The British Association of the Hard of Hearing
7-11 Armstrong Road
London W3 7JL   01-743 1110

The British Deaf Association
38 Victoria Place
Carlisle CA1 1HU   (Carlisle) 0228 48844

The English Deaf Chess Association
41 Frederick Street
Brighton BN1 4AT

British Deaf Sports Council
see The British Deaf Association

Link, the British Centre for Deafened People
19 Hartfield Road
Eastbourne BN21 2AR   (Eastbourne) 0323 638230

British Tinnitus Association
105 Gower Street
London WC1E 6AH   01-387 8033

National Association of Laryngectomee Clubs
39 Ecclestone Square
London SW1V 1PP   01-834 2857

Marie Curie Memorial Foundation
28 Belgrave Square
London SW1X 8QG   01-235 3325
(will hire out suction equipment)

Disabled Living Foundation
380–384 Harrow Road
London W9 2HU   01-289 6111

Health Education Council
78 New Oxford Street
London WC1A 1AH   01-637 1881

Index